NATURAL REMEDIES FOR ALLERGIES

SAFE SELF-HELP MEASURES FOR TREATING A WIDE RANGE OF MODERN ALLERGIES

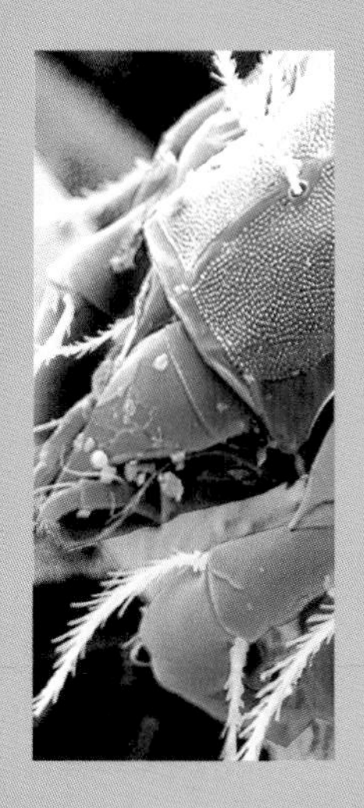

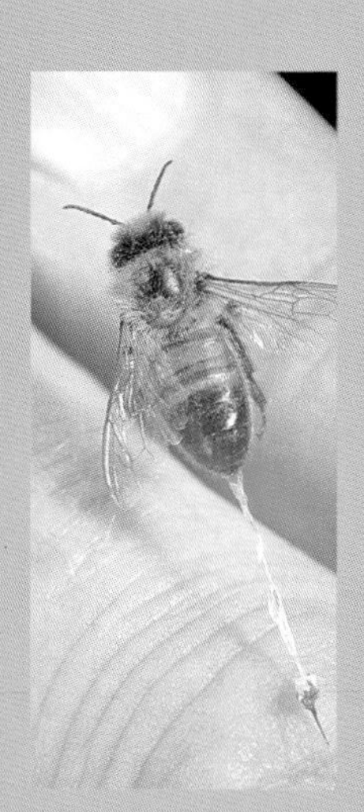

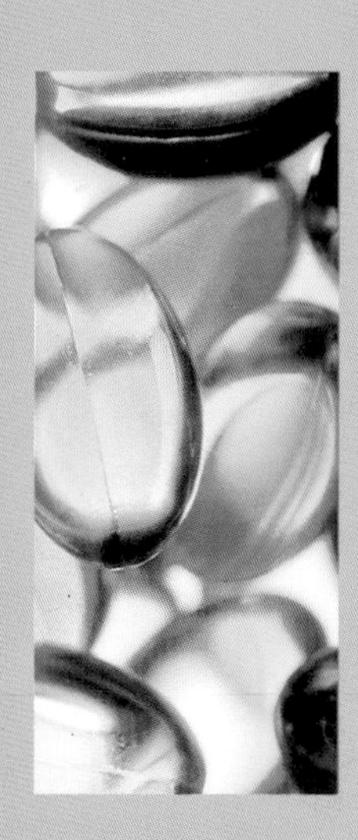

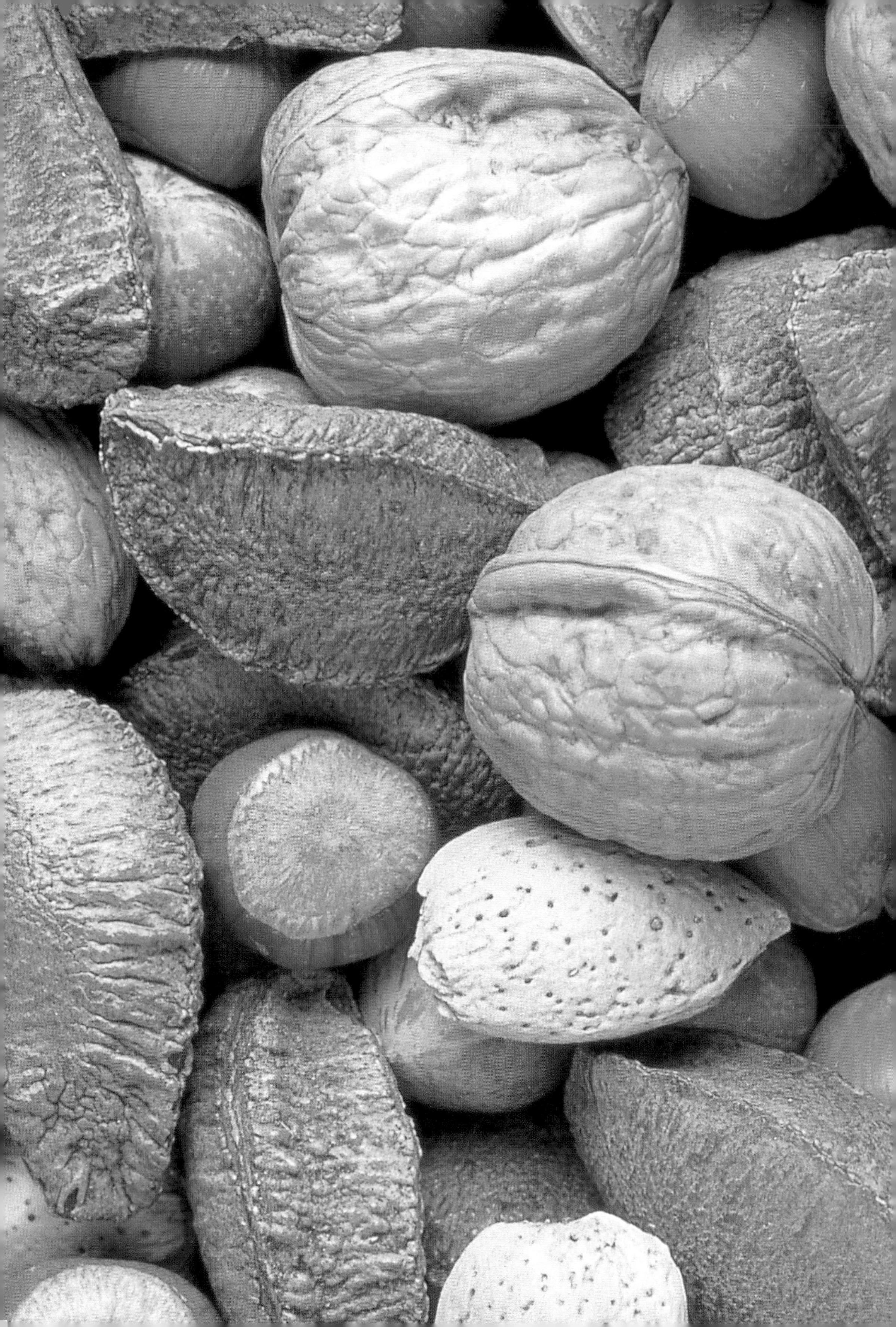

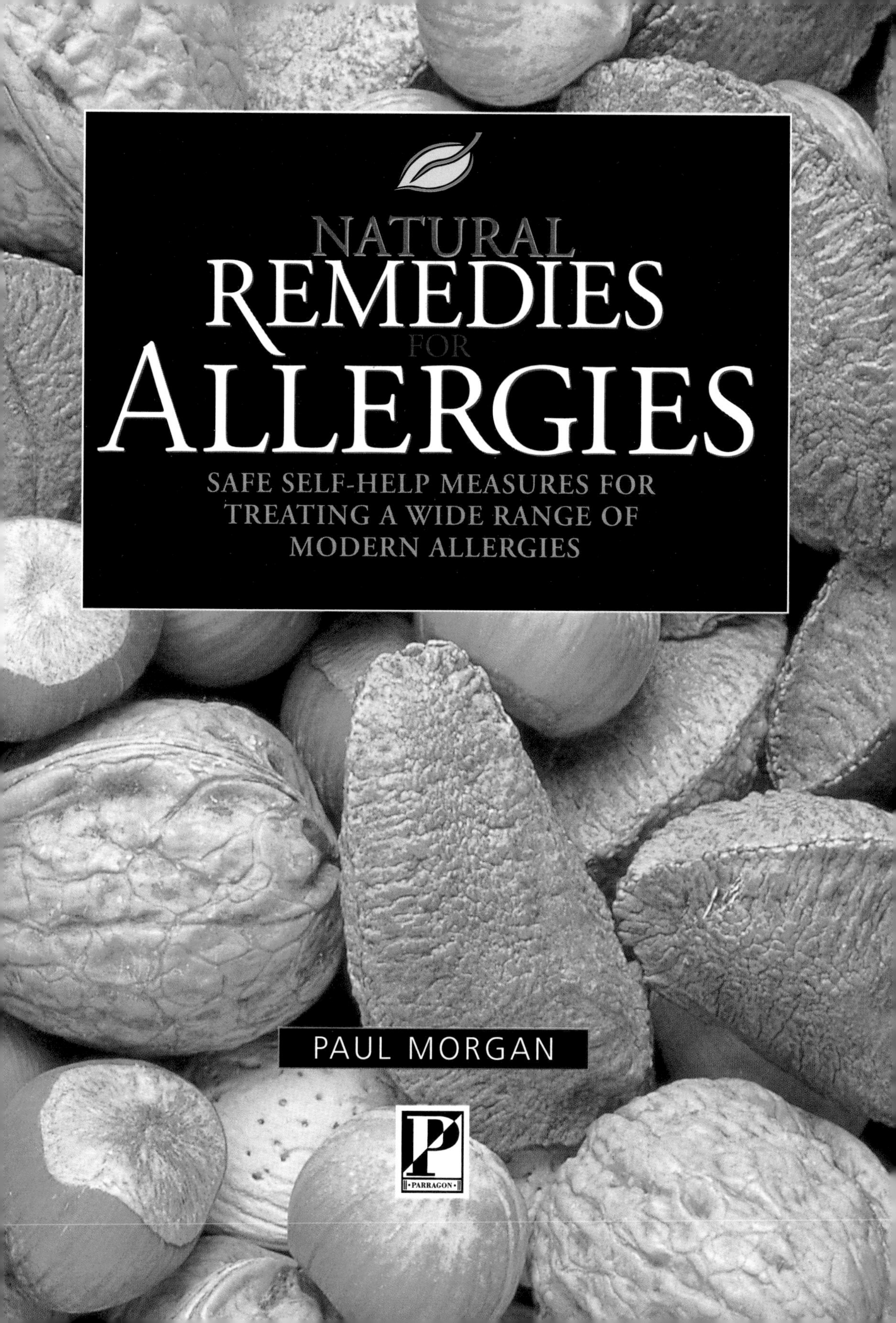
NATURAL
REMEDIES
FOR
ALLERGIES
SAFE SELF-HELP MEASURES FOR
TREATING A WIDE RANGE OF
MODERN ALLERGIES
PAUL MORGAN
PARRAGON

First published in 1998 by
Parragon
Queen Street House
4 Queen Street
Bath BA1 1HE

This edition reprinted in 1999

ISBN: 0-75253-176-X

Produced by Haldane Mason, London

Acknowledgements
Art Director: Ron Samuels
Editorial Director: Christopher Fagg
Designer: Zoë Mellors
Illustrator: Stephen Dew
Picture Research: Charles Dixon-Spain

Printed in Spain

Picture acknowledgements
Dyson: 118 , **The Garden Picture Library:** Brigitte Thomas 1, 5,100, 123 **Mary Evans Picture Library:** 7, **National Medical Slide Bank** 49, **Parragon:** 60, 61, 62, 63, 65, 76, 77, 78, 79,80,81, 83 84 **The Science Photo Library:** 38 (Left), 44, 45, 56, 66, 105,Tony Craddock 2–3, Erika Craddock 54, CC Studio 10, Alex Grey 11,Andrew Syred 1, 5,10, 15, E. Guetto 14, Dr P. Marazzi 17, Gary Watson 11, 19, Dr Jeremy Burgess 1, 5, 22, 47, 52 Saturn Stills 23, Mark Clarke 27, 43, Tek Image 29, Ricardo Arias 30, Ricardo Arias, Latin Stock 32 John Bavosi 34, Alfred Pasieka 35, Simon Fraser 36, Damien Lovegrove 37, 41, Bo Veisland, MI&I 38 (Right), Nasa 51, Seth Joel 59, Tim Malyon and Paul Biddle 72, Mark de Fraeye 75, BSIP, Collet 85.**Touchstone:** 86, 89, 91,95,97, 98, 99,

Every effort has been made to trace the copyright holders and we apologize in advance for any unintentional omissions. We would be pleased to insert the appropriate acknowledgement in any subsequent edition of this publication.

Parts of this book also appear in *Natural Remedies for Hayfever*, published by Parragon

IMPORTANT

The information, recipes and remedies contained in this book are generally applicable and appropriate in most cases, but are not tailored to specific circumstances or individuals. The author and publishers cannot be held responsible for any problems arising from the mistaken identity of any plants or remedies, or the inappropriate use of any remedy or recipe. Do not undertake any form of self diagnosis or treatment for serious complaints without first seeking medical advice. Always seek professional medical advice if symptoms persist.

Contents

The history of allergies

The first written reference to allergic reactions comes from ancient Greece, where Hippocrates, often regarded as the father of medicine, noted in his *Hippocratic Corpus* that some foods, such as cow's milk, caused stomach upsets and hives in some people but not in others. But – apart from the observation by Lucretius, the Roman poet, that 'one man's meat is another man's poison' – nothing much was heard on the subject of allergy for some six centuries. Then Galen, the most famous doctor of the age, noted in the second century AD that some people had adverse reactions to certain plants.

One Leonardo Botallo took up the story in 1565, giving the name 'rose cold' to the catarrh and asthma that a few people suffer when they are near blooming roses, and London doctor John Bostock christened the seasonal nose irritation from which he suffered 'Bostock's summer catarrh' – in fact it was hayfever.

The threads of the story were still coming together extremely slowly, but the pace picked up in the 1870s, when Wilhelm Dunbar, a German researcher, proved that pollen was responsible the for Bostock's condition. The problem was that nobody knew how pollen caused the problem. The breakthrough came when Charles Richet, Professor of Physiology at the University of Paris, became bored while he was on a tropical cruise with the then Prince of Monaco in 1902.

NEPTUNUS: A FINE, BIG DOG

Richet remembered some experiments he had performed a few years earlier, in which dogs injected with blood serum taken from eels suffered worse symptoms after repeated injections. So he started injecting dogs with poison taken from the jellyfish that surrounded the yacht. One dog – 'a fine, big dog by the name of Neptunus' – seemed perfectly happy after the first injection. After the second injection, however, Neptunus died.

Richet had discovered, albeit by cruel means, that a substance might be only moderately toxic when the body first encountered it but lethal when it was next met. Later, he found that this was not only true of poisons, but also of everyday substances, many of which could trigger a reaction to some degree. He had discovered the principle of allergy – though the term was coined by an Austrian paediatrician, Clemens von Pirquet, who combined two Greek words: *allos* ('different' or 'changed') and *ergos* ('work' or 'action').

Allergies were now firmly on the medical map, and work continued throughout the century to identify their precise mechanisms. But it was not until the mid-1970s that scientists were finally able to explain how an allergen works.

ONE IN FOUR PEOPLE

While the scientists pondered and experimented, however, the general public was becoming increasing aware of allergies in general, and of hayfever – also known as 'allergic rhinitis' – in particular. When Bostock had originally named his 'summer catarrh', the condition had been extremely rare. He commented that it had not 'been noticed as a specific affection until within the last ten or twelve years.' At the time, it seemed to be confined exclusively to the very well-to-do, though by the 1870s it had spread to the middle classes. Dr Charles Blackley, who specialized in researching and treating hayfever, noted that it seemed to affect only educated and professional people. Hayfever was not to maintain this exclusivity, however, for by the early 1900s, it was a common complaint among all classes.

And, just as the incidence of hayfever, perhaps the most common of all allergies, has continue to rise in a remarkable fashion – to the point that today one in six teenagers is affected – so allergies in general have become more and more common. It is impossible to be precise, but the generally accepted estimate is that about 25 per cent of the population is affected by an allergy of one type or other, and the figure continues to rise. Why? Nobody knows, though there are theories in plenty – all of them, however, remain unproved.

THE ALTERNATIVE PATH

This general sense of uncertainty is not confined to questions about the incidence of allergies but to their medical treatment as well. In the short term pills and potions can help to relieve symptoms, but only at the risk of side-effects. In the long term, conventional medicine has few answers to the problem. So people are increasingly turning to alternative remedies: to more natural ways of treating allergic reactions and of reducing their risk by a combination of holistic therapies and down-to-earth preventive measures. And the purpose of this book is to help you do just that.

Charles Richet (1850–1935), Professor of Physiology at the University of Paris, was the founder of scientific allergy studies.

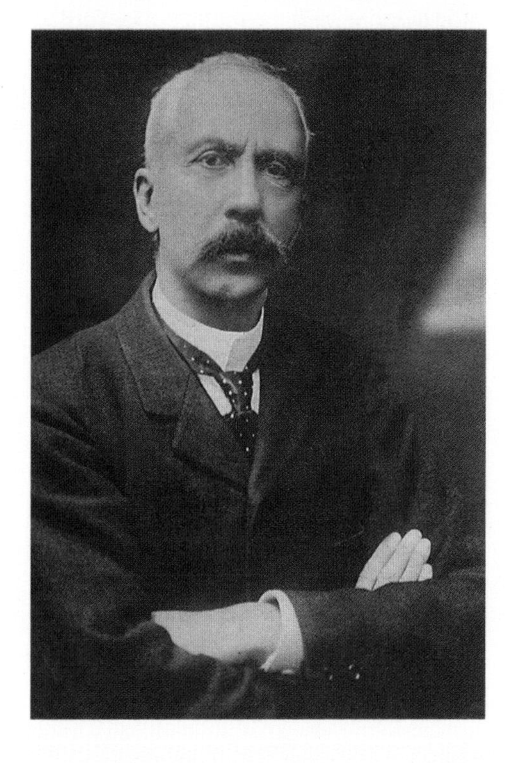

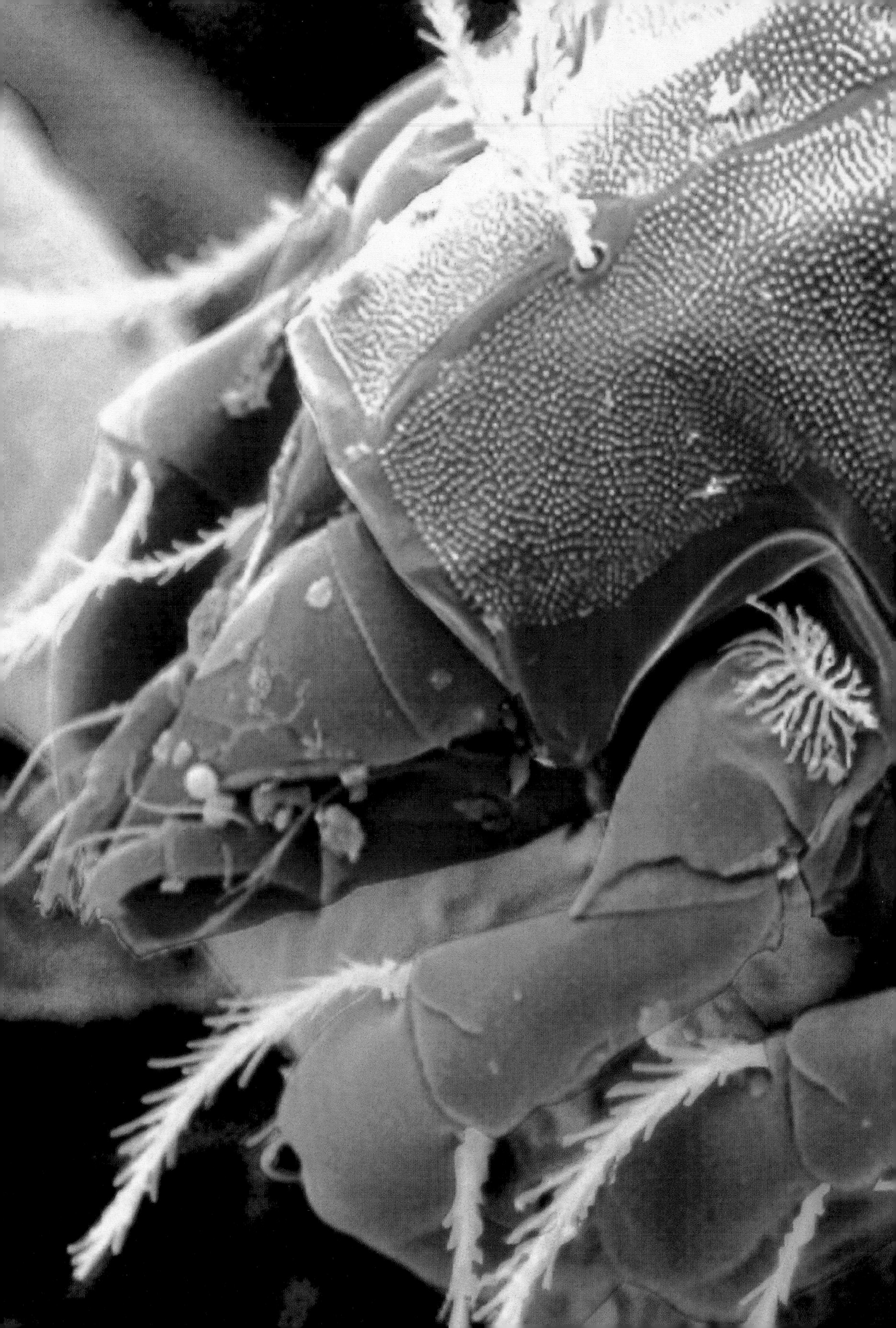

CHAPTER 1

Allergies
and conventional medicine

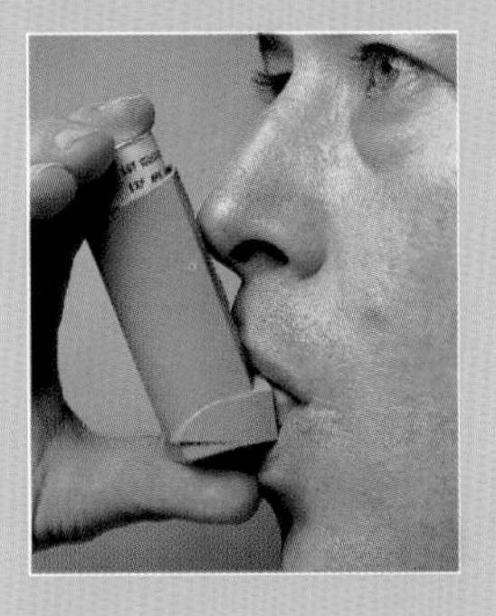

'Forewarned is forearmed' – something of a cliché, but none the less true for all that. An understanding of the mechanism that causes an allergic reaction as well as of the ways in which cross-reactions occur will help you devise strategies for avoiding allergens and also alert you to the types of natural remedy which may be effective in your particular case.

So in this section of the book you will find out what an allergy is, what types of allergy there are, what the symptoms of an allergic reaction are and how conventional medicine tries to deal with these symptoms and to prevent allergic reactions in the first place.

WHAT IS AN ALLERGY? • WHAT CAUSES AN ALLERGY? • CROSS-REACTIONS • CONVENTIONAL MEDICAL TREATMENTS

What is an allergy?

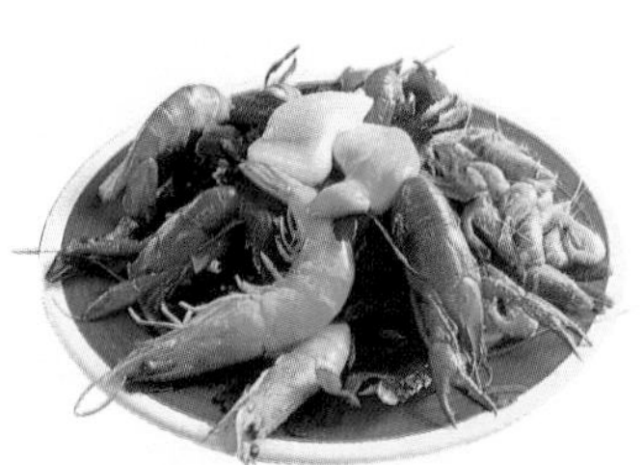

It's easy enough to say that you are allergic to something, whether it be pollen (as in hayfever), shellfish or milk, to give some common examples. In fact, however, the statement conceals an extremely complex sequence of reactions and events that take place in your body, both on your first exposure to something to which you become allergic and on subsequent exposures to it. And in order to understand how the sequence unravels, you have to understand something of the workings of the immune system, the body's natural defence mechanism against foreign invaders.

It is somewhat misleading to think of the immune mechanism as something as defined as a 'system', because in fact it is a response that takes place throughout the body. A clear fluid, lymph, seeps out of the blood into a network of vessels that form the lymphatic system, carrying with it millions of specialist 'immune' cells, to bathe all the cells in the body.

ANTIBODIES

Among these immune cells are chemicals called antibodies. The human body creates vast numbers of these soon after birth. Each antibody is able to recognize a specific type of chemical from a range of harmful substances called 'antigens'. When an antibody recognizes an antigen it sticks to it and acts as a marker, so that other defensive cells can find it and destroy it. At the same time, the body starts to mass-produce further quantities of the same antibody to deal with future threats. (This is the principle of immunization, whereby the body's production of antibodies is stimulated to combat particular invaders.)

Antibodies mark antigens in different ways. Some markers attract immune cells which work gently over a long period of time, without any symptoms; but others attract special immune cells, called mast cells, neutrophils and basophils, which rapidly release potent chemicals – such as histamine, also found in stinging nettles – in order to destroy the offending antigens quickly and completely. In the latter case, the markers are chemicals known as imunoglobulin E or IgE.

Histamine has a number of effects of which the most obvious is inflammation: the small blood vessels, the capillaries, dilate, and more fluid seeps from them into the surrounding tissues, so that there is an increase in the amount of lymph fluid in the area. But this also acts as a signal for more mast cells to join in the fight and release further chemicals, and more and more antibodies that are specific to the antigen are produced – so the exercise is self-perpetuating, until the invader has been destroyed and the body is safe.

TOO MANY MARKERS

The problem arises when the body becomes confused between what is potentially harmful and what is harmless. In cases of allergy, antibodies react as if a harmless substance is harmful – this substance is treated as an antigen, and is called an 'allergen'.

Why the body decides that a substance is an allergen remains a mystery, though a genetic factor is known to be involved (see pp. 12–13). But we do know that the severity of an individual's response to an allergen depends on how many IgE markers are present in his or her body. The more there are, the more mast cells are attracted and the more chemicals are released, which causes more inflammation and makes the symptoms of an allergic reaction worse.

SENSITIZATION

Sometimes – as in hayfever – an allergen produces a similar response each time someone is exposed to it: the results are unpleasant but are not particularly dangerous. At other times, an allergen can trigger another condition – such as asthma – which may be dangerous to the victim if the level of exposure is high or the response is severe. But the greatest danger to life comes from a phenomenon known as 'sensitization' – and it is this that killed Charles Richet's dog, Neptunus (see pp. 6–7).

In this phenomenon, the body becomes sensitized to an allergen on its first exposure to it. There are no particular symptoms at this time, but the body has responded to the allergen by producing huge quantities of antibodies. The second time that the allergen is encountered, these attract vast quantities of mast cells, which, in turn, release enormous quantities of histamine. The result can be that the body goes into shock – anaphylaxis (see pp. 24–5) – and immediate medical attention is necessary, otherwise the result can be fatal.

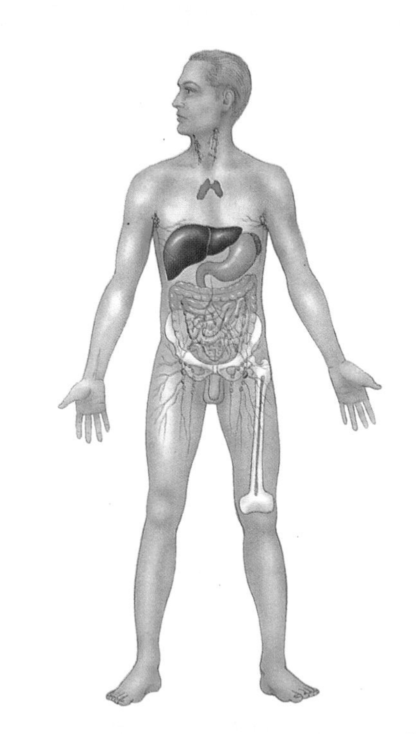

The human lymphatic system (in green) carries immune cells to all parts of the body via nodes in the armpits and groin.

What causes an allergy?

The short answer, unsatisfactory though it may be, is that nobody knows precisely what causes an allergy. However, two factors are known to have some influence over whether an allergy develops. The first of these is heredity – a tendency to allergies runs in families, so it is suspected that there is some genetic component to allergies that is not yet known. The second factor is psychological, and emotional pressures, such as stress, can trigger an allergic reaction.

THE GENETIC CONUNDRUM

About a third of people have IgE levels that are sufficiently high to cause allergies. Such people are said to be 'atopic', but not all atopic people develop allergies – as few as one in three actually do so – and it is common for several members of a family to be atopic but for only one or two of them to display allergic symptoms. Clearly, the development of an allergy is not a matter of simple inheritance and must involve a malfunction in several aspects of the immune system.

Even so, there is still a 30–35 per cent chance that a child will develop an allergy if one parent has an allergy – whatever it may be – and a 50–60 per cent chance if both parents have allergies. And as one child in six develops an allergy, even when there is no family history, the chances of developing an allergy are doubled in the first case and quadrupled in the second.

The question is: 'Which allergy will it be?' It is slightly more likely that the allergy will be to pollen rather than to anything else and will result in hayfever, but it could be to peanuts or to cow's milk. Even then, allergies can change – it is not uncommon for children to lose one allergy as they grow up, only to become allergic to something else. (A factor thought to have some effect here lies in the antigens to which children are exposed, and by which they become sensitized, in early life.)

One theory explaining why the incidence of allergies is rising so fast in the West while allergies are rare in the Third World is that the hygiene and vaccinations that are part of modern life in developed countries leave the immune system with little to do. As a result, it over-reacts, turning aggressive mast cells against minor irritants rather than the serious infections they were designed to combat.

PSYCHOLOGICAL FACTORS

Some people reject the notion that psychological factors are involved in the majority of medical conditions – they think they are being told: 'It's all in the mind.' Yet it's true that stress – worry, mental and emotional pressure, call it what you will – plays an important part in both the cause of numerous medical problems, including allergies, and the human body's response to them.

One study has shown that children of quick-tempered, aggressive, emotionally closed and over-protective parents suffer more allergic reactions, with worse symptoms, than children who live in a calm, peaceful home environment. To appreciate why this should be so, it's important to understand how the stress reaction works.

THE MECHANICS OF STRESS

It is only in recent times, in terms of our evolutionary history, that human beings have not had to live their daily lives under the threat of extreme physical danger. As a result, we retain the primitive systems that enabled early humans to survive, and these can be summed up in the 'fight or flight' reaction. Essentially, this means that danger triggers an immediate response by the involuntary or autonomic nervous system – that is, the response is made without conscious thought. Stress hormones – adrenaline being one of the most important – flood the body, preparing it for decisive physical action.

Modern life, especially urban life, produces daily stress events. The 'fight or flight' response is also triggered, though at a lower level, by emotional stress, so stress hormones are ever-present in the body, thereby raising blood pressure, increasing muscular tension and maintaining high levels of blood sugar.

As far as allergies are concerned, this has two effects. The first is that the adrenal glands, which produce adrenaline, are working full-time and are unable to produce sufficient extra adrenaline to fight the histamine released by mast cells (see pp. 10–11). The second effect relies on the fact there are two parts to the autonomic nervous system: the sympathetic system, which primarily controls the stress response; and the parasympathetic system, which deals with the immune response and the fight against infection. If the autonomic system as a whole is constantly active, the immune response – and in particular the part of it that does not rely on the aggressive mast cells – is likely to suffer.

It is for this reason that some of the remedies discussed in the third section of this book are concerned with reducing stress and emphasizing a positive approach to dealing with the symptoms of allergies.

POTENTIAL ALLERGENS

There are four main types of allergen, but which one you are allergic to seems to depend mainly on chance. They are:

- *the substances we eat and drink, called 'ingestants': examples include peanuts, shellfish and penicillin;*
- *the substances we touch, called 'contactants': example include latex gloves and primula leaves;*
- *substances injected into the body, such as insulin and, again, penicillin;*
- *substances that are inhaled, called 'inhalants': examples include pollen and dust mite droppings.*

Cross-reactions

We have looked at how antibodies recognize allergens, but it would be a mistake to think that they are so discriminating that they can identify an individual allergen with complete precision. In fact, recognition is based on fairly broad characteristics, which is just as well, because it means that the body can recognize antigens if they mutate into a slightly different form – as bacteria, for example, often do. The trouble is that this ability means that when large amounts of antibodies are produced to combat one substance, they may start to recognize another substance as an allergen, too. This second reaction is known as a 'cross-reaction'.

DUST MITE DROPPINGS AND KIWI FRUIT

Most cross-reactions are fairly harmless. For example, many hayfever sufferers are sensitive to ragweed pollen, and experience a cross-reaction when they come into contact with pollen from other members of the daisy family (*Compositae*). The result is an attack of hayfever, uncomfortable but not dangerous.

Ragweed pollen: much associated with hayfever.

However, there can also be cross-reactions to foods, as well as to other substances, such as cosmetics, the chemicals in hair shampoo, flakes of animal skin and house-dust mite droppings. On occasions, these can seem almost bizarre: one known cross-reaction is between dust mite droppings and kiwi fruit. Again, these cross-reactions are hardly ever dangerous, but on very rare occasions they can lead to anaphylactic shock (see pp. 24–5), which is an extremely serious problem. Generally, however, they are confined to tingling and itching around the mouth, in the case of a cross-reaction to food, an outbreak of hives (see pp. 44–5) or a tightness in the chest.

CALL FOR HELP

Most people who have allergies already know whether they are susceptible to cross-reactions and take appropriate measures to avoid whatever it may be that causes them. Generally, the only real danger comes if you are suffer from asthma (see pp. 34–6). If you are asthmatic, pay very close attention if you feel any tingling or swelling in your mouth after eating food, and make sure that you are in a position to call for help straightaway should your condition deteriorate.

Minute house-dust mites thrive in the home, where they scavenge on microscopic flakes of human skin and other detritus. Their droppings cause a range of allergic reactions.

PRECAUTIONS AGAINST CROSS-REACTIONS

As a general rule, allergic cross-reactions are mild and harmless, and there is no need to take any particular trouble to avoid any food or other substance that may have given rise to mild symptoms. However, you should make sure that you avoid altogether any substance that may be causing a cross-reaction in the following circumstances:

- *if the symptoms have ever been serious or you have had difficulty in breathing;*
- *if you suffer from asthma;*
- *if any symptoms become worse each time that you come into contact with a substance;*
- *if you are taking any medication – consult your doctor;*
- *if any symptoms appeared after eating peanuts, or anything made from peanuts (see pp. 30–3).*

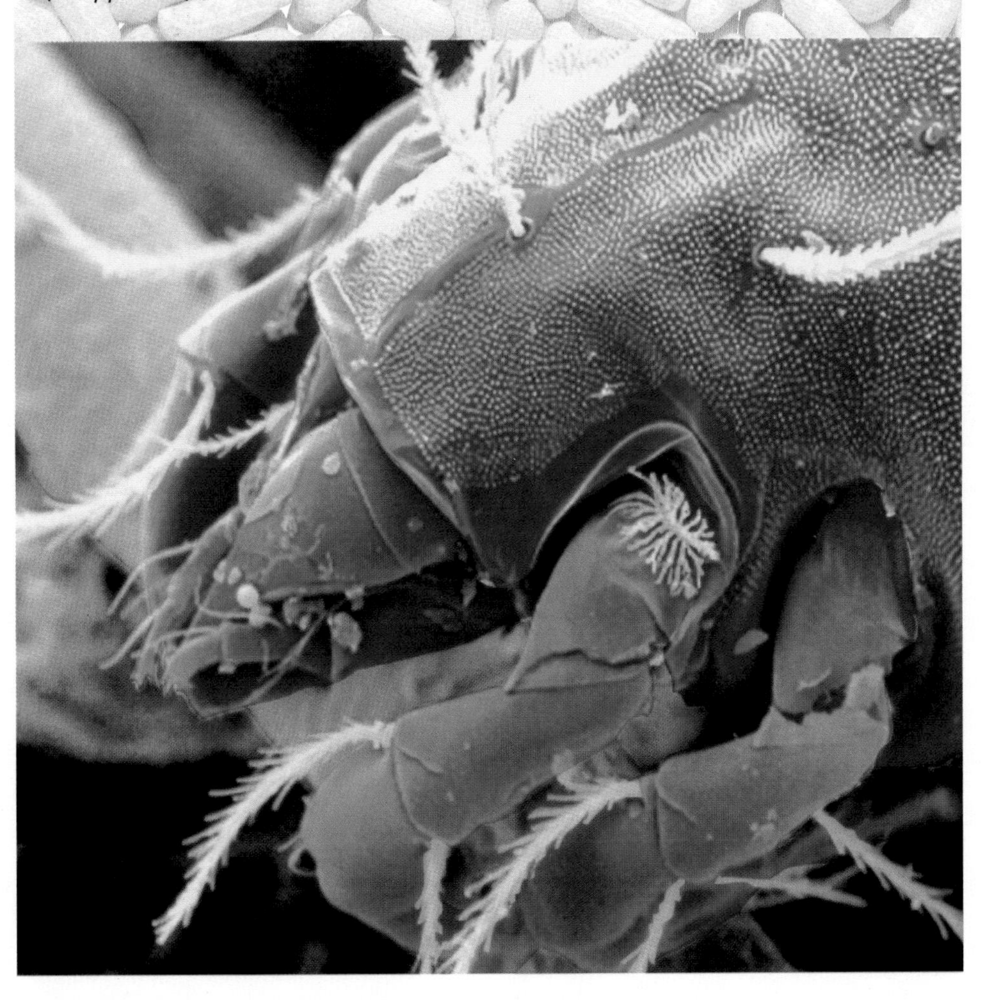

Conventional medical treatments

Since the detailed mechanism of how allergic reactions work is still not fully understood, conventional medical treatments generally aim to relieve symptoms by the use of drugs rather than to effect a lasting cure. Here we describe how these drugs work and what their side-effects can, on occasions, be. The intention is not to dissuade you from taking any such drugs – and you should certainly take them if they have been prescribed by your doctor.

The only medical alternative to drugs is desensitization treatments, which are time-consuming and not without their dangers. As far as short-term remedies are concerned, the drugs used fall into four categories, which are used singly or in combination. They are antihistamines, sympathomimetics, corticosteroids and mast cell stabilizers. In the case of asthma, bronchodilators, theophylline and anticholinergic agents are used as well.

ANTIHISTAMINES AND SYMPATHOMIMETICS

Since it is histamine, released by the mast cells (see pp. 10–11), that causes most of the symptoms in many allergic reactions, and in hayfever in particular, it would seem to make absolute sense to counter the effects of histamine with a drug specifically designed for that purpose. And antihistamines, which work by elbowing histamine molecules aside from receptors to which they would otherwise bind, certainly do the job effectively – though they have no impact on a blocked nose. You can buy them over the counter at most pharmacy stores, and if you are a hayfever sufferer it is often helpful if you take a course of them just before the pollen season.

The trouble is that antihistamines have their downside, too. Some of the older types of histamine can, as is well known, make you feel drowsy, but there are also

MEDICAL WATCHPOINT

Do not take antihistamines if:

- *it is essential that you drive;*
- *you are taking any other medication and have not asked your doctor whether it is wise to take them;*
- *you have any heart or circulatory problems or have high blood pressure;*
- *you have any liver, kidney or urinary problems.*

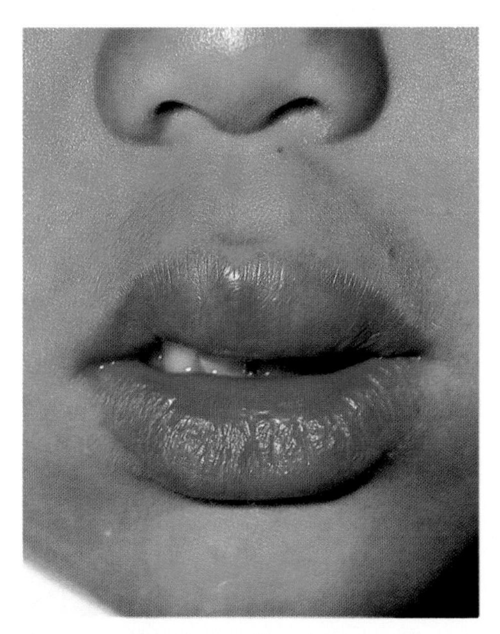

A severe allergic reaction to peanuts. When serious symptoms develop quickly, seek immediate medical advice.

possibilities of dizziness, tremors and blurred vision – for this reason, you should never drive while taking antihistamines. This is less of a problem with the most recent generation of antihistamines, but the problem exists nevertheless. In addition, antihistamines should not be taken in a number of other circumstances, the most important of which are listed on the page opposite.

Sympathomimetics mock the action of adrenaline, which counteracts histamine naturally inside the body. These drugs, many of which can be bought without prescription, are normally taken in the form of nose or eye drops, and they are effective at dealing with inflammation – acting like adrenaline, they force the blood vessels to contract, so reducing the swelling. Again, unfortunately, there is a hitch: first, adrenaline is one of the stress hormones, so sympathomimetics can induce the 'flight or flight' reaction (see pp. 12–13) to some degree, with all this entails; second, if they are taken for longer than a few weeks, the tissues become accustomed to them and larger doses will be necessary – but these will increase the side-effects.

To give the benefits of both types of drugs – but also the potential problems – antihistamines and sympathomimetics are sometimes both included in the same preparations. These can be bought without precription, and come in the form of either liquid or tablets.

CORTICOSTEROIDS

One of the main problems caused by allergies is that of inflammation, and

MEDICAL WATCHPOINT

Do not take sympathomimetics, either on their own or in combination with antihistamines, if:

- *you have heart or circulatory problems or high blood pressure;*
- *you are pregnant, trying to become pregnant or are breast-feeding;*
- *you have epilepsy;*
- *you are taking any other medication and have not asked your doctor whether it is wise to take them.*

corticosteroids are anti-inflammatory drugs that mimic the effect of cortisol, a hormone that is produced naturally by the body. They are powerful drugs and must be prescribed by a doctor, but they work effectively and can be given in a variety of ways. The most common of these is in the form of nose drops, though corticosteroid eye drops can alleviate conjunctivitis. The drugs can also be given in the form of tablets, injections or inhalants. Hayfever sufferers may be given a single, slow-release injection that lasts for the whole hayfever season, while asthmatics use corticosteroid inhalers as a preventive against the onset of asthma, although these drugs are not used to treat an asthma attack in progress.

This time the catch is that cortisol, which corticosteroids mimic, has a significant effect on the chemical balance of the body, and corticosteroids can add to this effect, to the detriment of this chemical balance. Another possibility is that the presence of artificial corticosteroids causes the body to produce less cortisol, with equally detrimental effects.

However, corticosteroid drugs are changed synthetically to boost the anti-inflammatory effect and reduce the effect on the body's chemistry, and it is fair to say – at least in the case of nose and eye drops – that any detrimental effect is minimal. Despite this, asthmatics are generally advised to inhale them for only a week at most. Problems are likely to arise only in the case of an extended course of tablets or a slow-release injection.

MAST CELL STABILIZERS

Corticosteroids themselves have a certain amount of success when it comes to stabilizing mast cells and reducing the amount of histamine that they release. Recently, several drugs have been developed that have this specific task, the best known of which is disodium cromoglycate (cromolyn sodium, or DSCG). These have no major side-effects, though there may be some passing irritation of the nasal membranes, and it is worth asking your doctor if you can try mast cell stabilizers. They are available as eye or nose drops, and can be bought over the counter. If you have hayfever, it is worth starting a course of mast cell stabilizers several weeks before the start of the pollen season; if you are an asthmatic, mast cell stabilizers taken daily may help prevent an asthma attack, although they cannot stop an asthma attack once one has started.

BETA ADRENERGIC BRONCHODILATORS

These drugs, of which there are many different types, are used solely to treat asthma attacks and their onset. They work by relaxing the smooth muscles in the walls of the bronchioles, the tiny air passages in the base of the lungs that constrict during an asthma attack (see pp. 34–7). Possible side-effects of these drugs include an increased heart rate, dizziness, nervous tension and, in some case, headaches, nausea and cramps. However, an asthma attack can be life threatening and, if your doctor has prescribed them, you should take bronchodilators if an asthma attack develops or you suspect one is imminent.

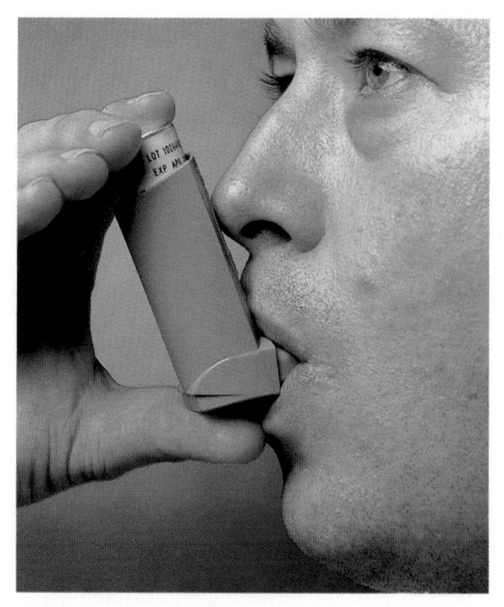

An asthma inhaler dilates tiny air passages in the lungs to prevent attacks.

THEOPHYLLINE

This chemical also relaxes the smooth muscle of the bronchioles and so is used in the treatment of asthma, often alongside bronchodilators. It is often used, too, to help prevent an attack of asthma during the night.

ANTICHOLINERGIC AGENTS

These drugs are sometimes used in the case of sudden, serious asthma attacks to help open up the airways. They are not generally used on a day-to-day basis.

DESENSITIZATION THERAPY

The only treatment that attempts a long-term cure for allergies such as hayfever, allergies to house-dust mite droppings and the venom of bees and wasps is desensitization therapy. There are three types: hyposensitization, enzyme-potentiated desensitization and neutralization.

Hyposensitization involves injecting a series of solutions of a given allergen beneath the skin. At first the solution is extremely dilute, but its strength is increased, week by week, over a period of ten weeks or so – the idea is to allow the body to learn to tolerate the allergen. This treatment has to be repeated for four or five years, so it is extremely time consuming. Nevertheless it is often successful. However, it is now extremely difficult to obtain this form of treatment outside of special centres, of which there are few, because there is a significant risk that those treated will develop anaphylactic shock and die. In practical terms, this form of treatment is virtually unavailable.

The second therapy is enzyme-potentiated desensitization (EPD), which is more widely available and is successful in around 50 per cent of cases. A collection of different allergens is mixed with a special enzyme – a chemical that can act as a catalyst to other chemical reactions – and injected beneath the skin to desensitize the body to the allergens. Treatment may have to be repeated each year – in the case of hayfever, for as long as five years.

Neutralization therapy relies on injecting allergens beneath the skin or placing drops of them in soluble form under the tongue. Various concentrations are used until no allergic reaction can be detected – this concentration is said to represent the patient's 'neutralizing dose'. A solution of this strength is made up, and the patient is asked to take two to three drops a day before any likely exposure to an allergen – as in the case of the pollen season and hayfever – reducing the dose thereafter.

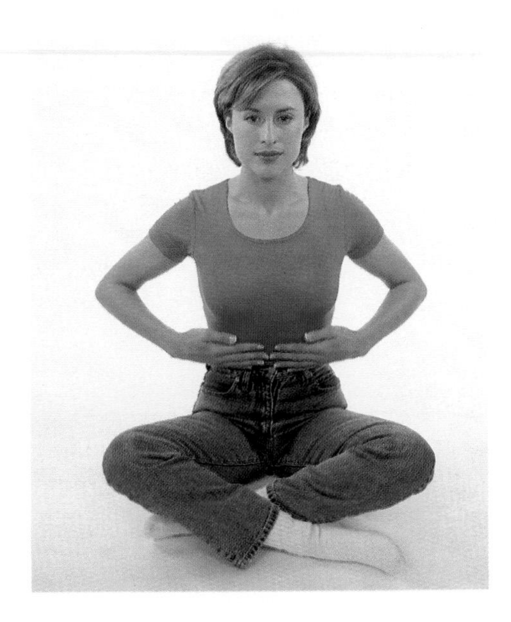

BREATHING DURING AN ASTHMA ATTACK

The difficulty in breathing that an asthma sufferer experiences during an attack can cause panic, and it is important that you learn how to control your breathing in order to cope with the problem when it arises. This technique is also useful if you feel any tightness of the chest during any other allergic reaction.

Sit in the position illustrated when practising, because this opens the rib-cage and expands the chest, so that less muscular effort is needed to breathe. Then relax your body.

Place both your hands on the lower edges of your ribs, with your fingers nearly touching. As you inhale, your fingers will move up and apart.

Breathe in deeply and smoothly through your nostrils and feel how your diaphragm moves out and down and your ribs expand up and out. Hold the breath for a few seconds, and then let the breath go, naturally and without force.

Repeat the exercise with your hand over the middle of your chest; then with your hands over your collar bones.

Once you have mastered this exercise you will have a better appreciation of the mechanism of breathing and how it can be controlled. Then you can put it into practice during an asthma attack or when your chest feels tight when you are experiencing an allergic reaction.

ALLERGIES AND EXERCISE

Doctors treating asthmatics or people with allergies that cause congestion or blockages of the nose, sinuses and airways, making it difficult for them breathe properly, often refer patients to a physiotherapist, who can suggest a course of remedial exercises, some of which are described below. However, it is unwise to start an exercise programme or to continue with an existing one without having consulted your doctor; this is especially important if you suffer from exercise-related asthma or have ever suffered from anaphylaxis (see pp. 24–5).

This time, however, sit straight in a chair with your arms over its back and try to control your breathing by means of the technique you have learned. You will find it helpful, but remember that it is an aid, and not a substitute for any medication that your doctor has prescribed for you to take in the event of an asthma attack.

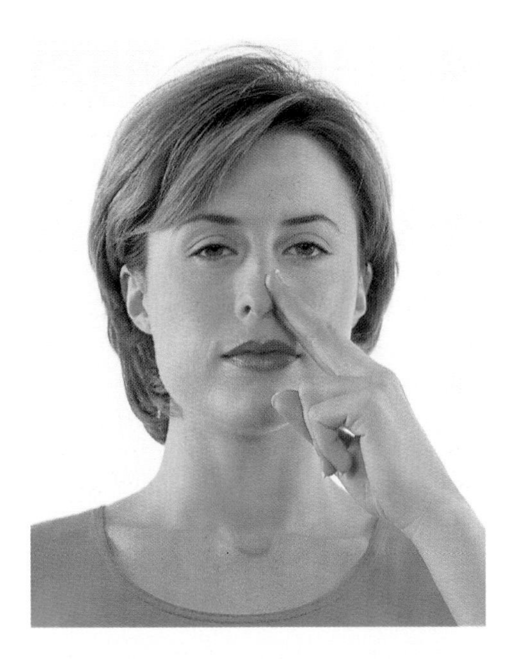

SUN AND MOON BREATHING

The basic movements of this technique, which comes from Eastern medicine, are similar to those in the basic technique on the opposite page, but the principle behind them is different. The sun and moon are seen as symbols of the positive and the negative: you inhale positive energy and exhale negative energy.

Sit in an upright chair and pinch your nostrils shut with one hand – use your thumb to close one nostril and a finger on the other. Breathe naturally through your mouth as you practise opening and shutting your nostrils by releasing the pressure of your finger and thumb.

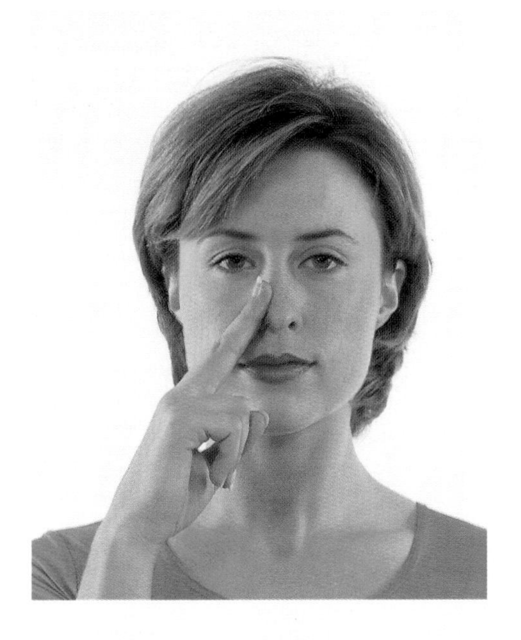

When you are confident, inhale deeply through your right nostril (as in the basic technique), keeping the left one shut. Hold this deep breath for the length of time that it took to inhale – this might be difficult at first – and then exhale through your left nostril, keeping the right nostril shut for a similar length of time: the timing ratio should be one part inhaling to one part breath-holding to one part exhaling (represented as the ratio 1:1:1). With much practise, adherents of the technique can achieve a ratio of 1:4:2, but 1:2:2 is sufficient to boost the flow of energy and calm the mind.

After five inhalations breathe through both nostrils, blank your mind and relax fully.

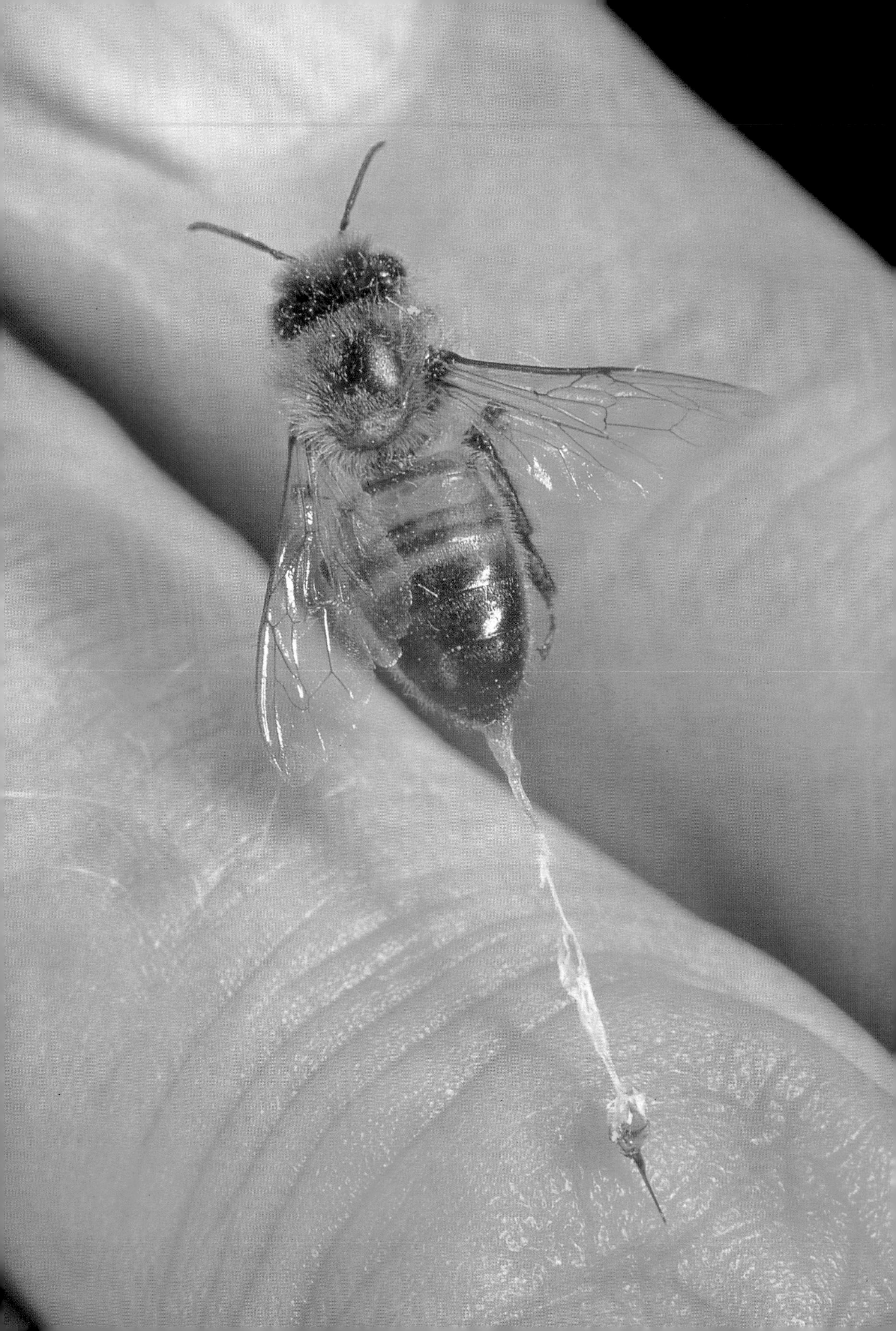

CHAPTER 2

Types of allergy

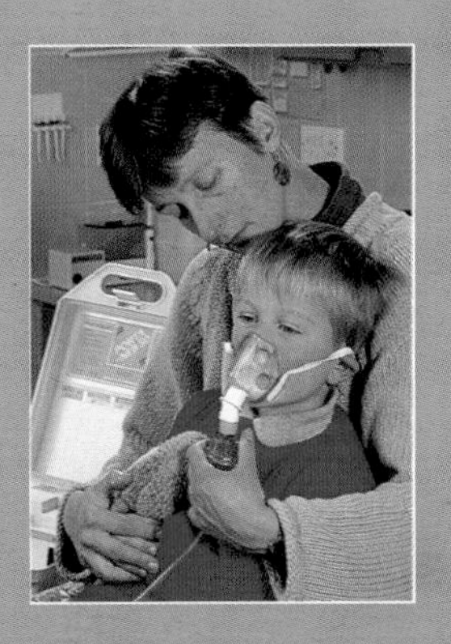

We've seen the nature of an allergic response and examined the mechanism that underlies it, so in this section of the book we're going to take a more detailed look at the various types of allergy that exist. One difficulty, however, is that many people refer to conditions that are not, in fact, based on any allergic reaction as allergies. For example, lactose intolerance (see pp. 30–1), which is an inability to digest milk that causes allergy-like symptoms, is not a true allergy because its cause is a deficiency of the enzyme lactase, which is needed to break down lactose, a sugar found in milk. For completeness, however, most types of allergy, whether true or false, are considered here.

ANAPHYLACTIC SHOCK • CHILDREN'S ALLERGIES

DRUG REACTIONS • FOOD ALLERGIES

ASTHMA • EAR AND EYE ALLERGIES • HAYFEVER

HIVES • INSECT STINGS

SKIN ALLERGIES

TOTAL ALLERGY SYNDROME

Anaphylactic shock

Anaphylaxis is the most extreme, and most dangerous, form of allergic reaction. Unlike most allergies, which involve a localized reaction to an irritant, anaphylaxis involves the whole body. There is a massive release of histamine, leading to swelling, fever and profound shock to the whole body. Anyone suffering from anaphylactic shock is in need of emergency treatment and should be taken to hospital immediately. Without treatment, anaphylaxis can be fatal.

Anaphylaxis is rare, but it is still a real danger to anyone who has an allergic condition. Like other forms of allergy, it depends on prior sensitization to a particular allergen. Often the initial reaction will be quite marked and should be taken as a warning sign that the next encounter with the allergen might produce the massive response of an anaphylactic attack.

WHAT HAPPENS IN ANAPHYLACTIC SHOCK?

The effects of anaphylaxis, as in other allergic reactions, are due to the release of histamine by the mast cells. The difference is that mast cells throughout the body, and not just at the site of irritation, are involved. Histamine dilates blood vessels and makes them more leaky. The body's blood supply suddenly has to occupy a much larger volume than before and, as a result, blood pressure falls to the point at which proper circulation can no longer be maintained. The pulse becomes weak and feeble, and there may be extreme pallor. At the same time, the bronchi – the passages supplying air to the lungs – become narrower and breathing becomes difficult. Asthma sufferers are particularly at risk when this happens.

The symptoms of anaphylaxis may appear rapidly – sometimes within a few minutes – or they may develop over an hour or two. The first signs are the itchiness of the nose, eyes and mouth that is characteristic of most allergic reactions. However, in this case, the lips and tongue are likely to swell up, obstructing breathing, and a 'lump' may develop at the back of the throat. The pulse will become weak. There may be abdominal pains, confusion and a feeling of anxiety or dread. The complete collapse of the circulatory and respiratory systems may follow, requiring urgent admission to hospital and the immediate use of resuscitation equipment.

WHAT CAUSES ANAPHYLACTIC SHOCK?

Almost anything can cause anaphylactic shock – it is the acute sensitivity of the body rather than the character of the allergen that determines whether anaphylaxis will occur. However, certain triggers appear to be responsible more often than others. Bee and wasp stings can set off anaphylaxis in sensitive people, as can allergies to particular foods.

In addition, anaphylactic shock is a hazard of hyposensitization treatment (see pp. 18–19). This technique is designed to accustom the body to an allergen by gradually subjecting it to larger and larger doses. In this way, the immune system becomes familiar with the allergen and ceases to treat it as an enemy. Unfortunately, the immune system sometimes fails to adjust to increasing exposure; it may not react to begin with, but after a while it may take sudden and violent exception to the continuing assault, and an anaphylactic shock is the result. There is usually some indication that this may happen – in the form of a mild, sometimes almost unnoticeable reaction to a previous treatment – and the allergist will be on the look out for such a reaction and will adjust the treatment accordingly.

THE RECOVERY POSITION

The recovery position is used to avoid the dangers that can occur during unconsciousness, and ensures that the airway is open and clear.

Kneeling to one side of the victim, turn his/her head towards you and tuck the arm nearest to you under the victim's body. Lay the other arm across the victim's chest and place the ankle furthest from you over the other ankle.

Grasping the clothing over the hip farthest from you, pull the victim on to his/her front, using your knees to support the body and your hand to protect the head as you do so. Push the victim's head back to ensure a clear airway and check his/her breathing.

On the side to which the victim's face is turned, bend the arm and leg into right angles (see below). Check the position is stable and and ensure the airway is clear. Do not leave the victim unattended and wait for professional help.

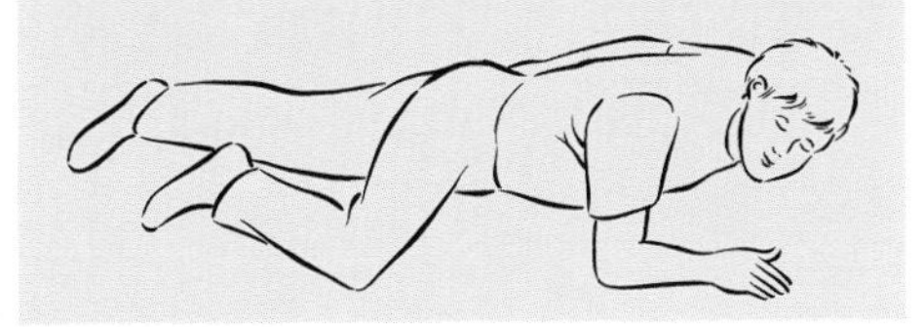

WHAT TO DO IN AN EMERGENCY

If you know or suspect that you are susceptible to anaphylactic shock, you should take the following precautions:

- *Always carry a syringe or inhaler containing adrenaline, which counters the effects of histamine in the tissues. Your doctor will be able to prescribe this for you.*
- *If you feel symptoms developing, go to a hospital immediately. Insist on being seen straight away, even if you have to barge to the head of a queue.*
- *If you have had an anaphylactic shock before and know what caused it (a particular type of food, for example), you should consider wearing a medical bracelet, available through your doctor or a pharmacist. If you are ever found unconscious, the information on the bracelet will help to get you the right treatment and could save your life.*

Children's allergies

Although allergies can develop at any age, they are far more likely to make their first appearance during childhood, and because babies and children are growing and developing, allergies that would have no long-term effects on an adult can do serious damage in an allergic child. The most common childhood allergic conditions are asthma and hayfever, but eczema and hives, food allergies and sensitivity to insect stings appear all too frequently as well. Parents with sensitive children should learn as much as they can about the particular condition concerned and learn also to recognize the signs and symptoms that identify an allergy in their child.

It can often be difficult to recognize an allergy in a baby or child. If your newborn has digestive problems, a chronic cough or skin rashes, are they the result of an allergy to antibodies in the mother's breast milk or are they due to mild bacterial or viral infection? Are your child's runny nose and sore throat signs of hayfever or simply the symptoms of a common cold?

IS YOUR CHILD ALLERGIC?

In the end, only your doctor or an allergist may be able to tell you if your child suffers from an allergy. But there are many things that you as a parent can do to help the diagnosis. First, you can check your own personal and family histories for evidence that allergic conditions 'run in the family'. A tendency to allergies is inherited, although many children who have the tendency will never actually become allergic (see pp. 12 –13). Second, you can take careful note of any pattern of symptoms, such as a rash, a runny nose or a cough, which tend to occur frequently. Check to see if the symptoms appear in similar circumstances every time – after eating a particular food or after contact with pets or with some particular type of bedding. Finally, take careful note of the frequency and duration of the symptoms as well their severity. It may be a good idea to keep a detailed diary of your child's symptoms

WARNING SIGNS

Be on the look out for the following symptoms, particularly if they become chronic or severe.

- *Red, itchy skin.*
- *Sneezing, runny nose and nasal congestion (hayfever).*
- *Wheezing, breathlessness or a recurrent cough (asthma).*
- *Red, watering eyes.*
- *Stomach pains, vomiting and diarrhoea (food allergies)*
- *Itchiness within the ears or a feeling that the ears are blocked.*
- *Constant itchiness of the roof of the mouth.*

(see pp. 102–103). If you decide to consult a doctor, the more information you can give the better. You will improve the chances of prompt and accurate diagnosis, and you will be able to take effective countermeasures more quickly.

PROBLEMS OF CHILDHOOD ALLERGIES

Allergies may cause problems at any age, but there are some problems that are particularly associated with allergies in childhood. Long-running congestion of the nose, for example, can lead to a child breathing through the mouth, particularly while asleep. The force of the air affects the way that the soft bones of the face develop, leading to distortions in the shape of the face and causing dental problems, which may require long periods of treatment.

Allergies that affect the ears can also have long-term effects. If a child's hearing is impaired while he or she is learning to talk, speech may not develop normally and learning can be affected. Some behavioural disorders, such as attention deficit disorder or hyperactivity may also be due to an allergy and normal childhood learning may be disrupted.

COPING WITH CHILDHOOD ALLERGIES

Allergic reactions can be frightening and confusing for a child – and also for the parents. The key advice is to remain calm and comforting. Your child needs to be able to put his or her trust in you, and panic on your part will only make matters worse.

MEDICAL ALERT

If some event – a wasp sting, for example – causes your child to swell up alarmingly, particularly in the throat, causing difficulty in breathing and swallowing, get help immediately. The child may be suffering from anaphylactic shock (see pp. 24–5). This is a real emergency, and the condition can be life-threatening.

If your child is suffering a bad asthma attack and the lips and the beds of the fingernails take on a bluish tinge, get to a hospital immediately. The child's body is being starved of oxygen, and his or her life is at risk.

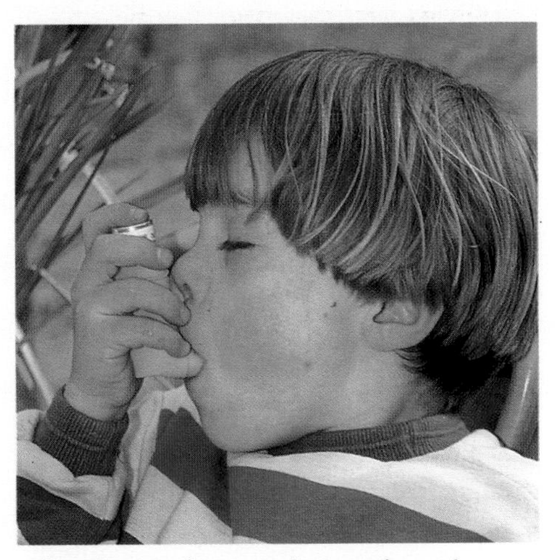

Allergic reactions, such as asthma, in childhood are alarming – but parents can learn to cope.

For the long-term control of childhood allergic conditions, you may need to follow the prevention and avoidance advice given on pp. 106–125. And for childhood asthma, breathing exercises (see pp. 20–21) can provide both comfort and relief.

Drug reactions

As many as one person in three will experience some form of adverse reaction to a drug. Usually, this takes the form of an unwanted side-effect, such as drowsiness, nausea or headache, and is simply a by-product of individual body chemistry. True drug allergy is less common, however, and can be difficult to recognize and identify. Nevertheless, some very common drugs – penicillin and aspirin, for example – are known to cause allergic reactions, and people who are sensitive should always be cautious when taking a new type of medication.

Drug reactions are something of a nightmare for the allergist. What looks like an allergy very often isn't one. A skin rash, for example, may seem to be caused by a drug, but is more often a symptom of the disease that the drug is intended to cure. In addition, drugs in the body are often broken down into many small chemical fragments, any or all of which may act as allergens.

Allergic symptoms may also be caused by psychological factors. Fainting or dizziness experienced in the dentist's chair, for example, may be caused by a fear of injections rather than an adverse response to the anaesthetic itself.

Rather surprisingly, drug allergies are also more common with drugs that are applied to the skin or injected than with those that are taken orally. When drugs are applied externally, the allergic reaction generally takes the form of contact dermatitis (see pp. 48–49). Suntan lotions, cosmetics, shampoos and other preparations can also cause allergic dermatitis.

COMMON DRUG ALLERGIES

While it can be difficult to be sure that an adverse drug reaction is due to an allergy, there are, nevertheless, some common drugs that are known to cause allergic reactions. Chief among these are penicillin, aspirin and, in the case of diabetics, insulin. All these drugs may cause reactions ranging from mild and inconvenient to catastrophic and life-threatening.

Penicillin usually causes a rash of pink to purplish spots on the arms, legs, back and chest. These normally disappear after two to three weeks and do not require treatment. On occasions, however, the reaction may be delayed and appear only around a week after treatment has begun. The symptoms of this delayed reaction can include fever, rash, joint pain, swollen lymph nodes and hives (urticaria). When they occur together, these symptoms are sometimes known as serum sickness because they can also be caused by the serum that is used in the preparation of certain vaccines.

TESTS AND CURES

As with other types of allergy, the offending allergen is usually identified by a skin prick test or a patch test (see pp. 104–105). A small quantity of the drug is dripped onto a small puncture in the skin or applied by means of an adhesive patch on the forearm or back. Any resulting inflammation is a sign of an allergic response.

Almost always, the best way to deal with a drug allergy is to avoid it: stop taking the drug and ask your doctor to prescribe an alternative. Always read the labels on proprietary medicines before buying them and learn which ingredients to avoid (see pp. 108–109). In very rare cases, it may not be possible to avoid a particular drug – aspirin is needed to treat some forms of juvenile rheumatoid arthritis, and penicillin or a related antibiotic may be vital for the treatment of serious bacterial disease. Insulin is essential for diabetics. In these cases, desensitization treatments are available (see pp. 18–19). Remember, though, that desensitization does not provide a permanent cure; its effects last for only as long as the treatment continues. If you need to take the drug in the future, you will have to undergo a fresh course of desensitization.

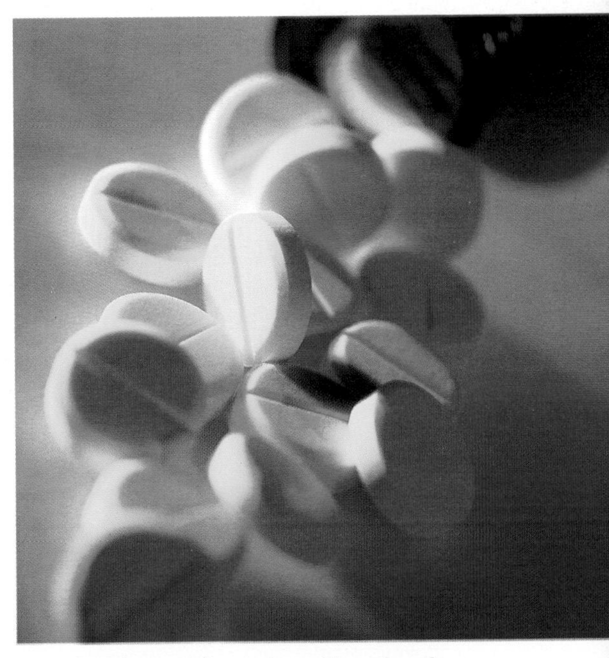

Aspirin, derived from the willow family, is a long-established pain reliever but may cause serious allergic reactions, particularly in children.

The reaction to aspirin usually causes the symptoms of hives. However, it may sometimes takes the form of the aspirin 'triad', which involves asthma, sinusitis and the formation of nasal polyps. Sensitivity to aspirin can also cause cross-reactions (see pp. 14–15) with another group of pain-killing drugs, known as non-steroidal anti-inflammatory drugs (NSAIDs), such as ibuprofen.

Aspirin should not be given to children under the age of 12 because of its association with a rare but potentially fatal disease known as Reye's syndrome. Paracetamol should be given instead.

If you are diabetic, you may well suffer from an allergy to insulin. This is usually mild, with redness and swelling round the site of the injection, which clears up after a short time. Occasionally, there is a more severe late-phase response (see p. 43), which occurs three or four hours after the injection, or a still later delayed response, which may take several days to clear up completely. Insulin allergy can often be cured quite simply by switching to a different form of insulin – from pork insulin to beef insulin, for example.

Food allergies

Food allergies are among the most intractable and mysterious of all the different types of allergy. The food we eat contains many thousands of different molecules, any one of which may provoke an allergic response in somebody, somewhere. The mere fact of feeling ill after eating a particular food does not necessarily indicate an allergy – you might think you are allergic to shellfish, for example, when in fact you are allergic to a particular agricultural chemical that has entered the water in the area where the shellfish were caught. People have been known to be allergic to chicken fed on one particular type of grain, but entirely at ease with chicken that have been fed on another.

Food allergies have been recognized since at least the time of the ancient Greeks. Some experts have even suggested that religious taboos about certain foods stem from a recognition that they have the potential to cause allergies. And mothers have long understood that there is a dietary component in many common conditions and complaints and have avoided giving certain types of food to their children.

Not all adverse reactions to food are due to allergy, however. The inability to digest milk, which produces allergy-like symptoms, is due to a deficiency of the enzyme lactase, which is needed to break down lactose, the sugar present in milk.

Bread is a prime source of essential carbohydrate, but a minority of people experiences a strong allergic reaction to the gluten in wheat.

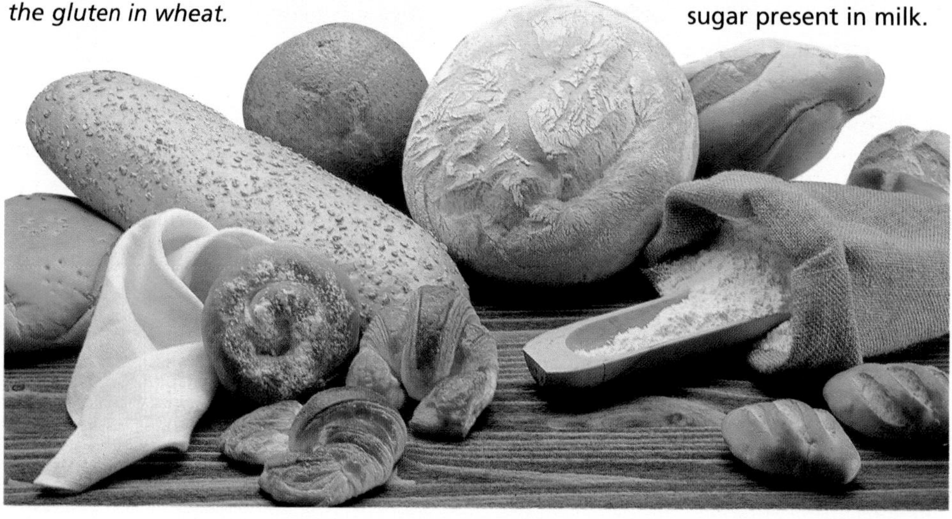

MEDICAL ALERT

If you experience any of the conditions or symptoms listed in the box (right) you should consult your doctor. There are many other potential causes besides food allergy, and if you try to treat them by adjusting your diet yourself, you may not get the treatment you need and the condition may get worse.

SYMPTOMS

Food allergy can affect almost any part of the body. In severe cases it can cause anaphylactic shock (see pp. 24–5), in which the whole body is involved. However, the most common symptoms are vomiting, nausea, diarrhoea and stomach cramps, which are often combined with asthma, eczema, hives, headache, earache and hayfever symptoms (runny nose, sneezing and watering eyes).

The whole subject of food allergy is complicated by the fact that a particular food will not always produce symptoms. They may appear only when there is some other factor at work – for example, your sensitivity may be increased by the presence of other allergens in your system. A bout of hayfever can produce a reaction to a type of food one day, even though you might have eaten it quite happily the day before. Psychological and emotional stress may also lead to the development of a food allergy, which is why relaxation techniques such as meditation, yoga and visualization which can relieve stress, are especially recommended for people who are susceptible to allergies.

CONDITIONS RELATED TO FOOD ALLERGIES AND INTOLERANCE

- Asthma
- Eczema (dermatitis)
- Hives (urticaria or nettle rash)
- Angioderma (a form of hives affecting deeper tissues of the body)
- Allergic rhinitis (hayfever)
- Sinusitis
- Migraine and other headaches
- Premenstrual syndrome
- Irritable bowel syndrome
- Crohn's disease and ulcerative colitis
- Peptic ulcers
- Gastritis
- Coeliac disease (gluten intolerance)
- Hypoglycaemia
- Complications of diabetes
- Rheumatoid arthritis
- Epilepsy
- Anxiety and depression
- Excessive fatigue
- Weight problems
- Racing heart-beat
- Childhood disorders (recurrent infections, attention deficit disorders, learning disorders)

The symptoms of food allergy can appear early in childhood, and experts suspect that food allergy is implicated in many childhood complaints, from attention deficit disorder (hyperactivity) to learning difficulties and from clumsiness to head-banging and other behavioural disorders. Similarly, there is evidence that food allergy has a part to play in many adult conditions (see table above). If there is a history of allergy in your family, you should note carefully if

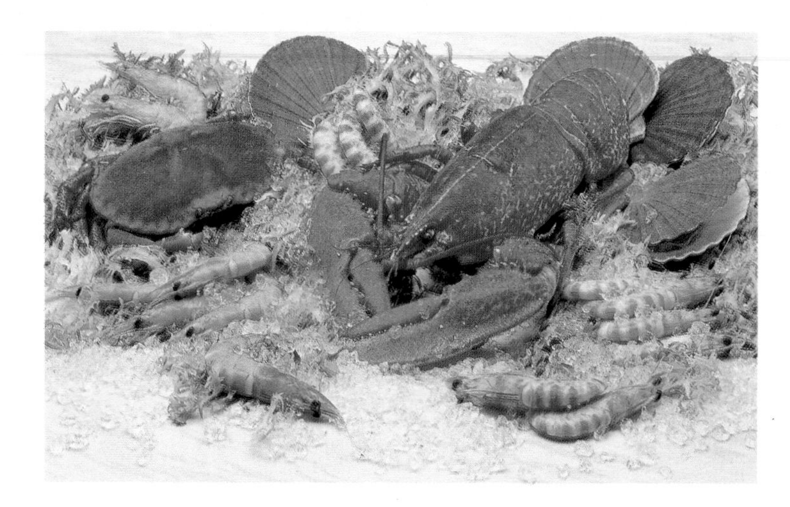

Seafood is well known for its often violent allergic effects. The most common culprits are shellfish.

there is any pattern in the appearance of your symptoms, and consult your doctor. Don't try to adjust your or your child's diet without medical advice – the problem may not be due to food allergy, and may need an entirely different form of treatment.

RECOGNIZING THE PROBLEM

As with other forms of allergy, food allergies require sensitization to the particular allergen or allergens involved. This often happens in infancy, and the initial symptoms are easily mistaken for something else – a cold, or excessive wind, for example. The early symptoms then disappear, but some time later – it may be days, months or years – they will reappear.

Even then, the symptoms of chronic food allergy can be difficult to recognize. In fact, food allergies are sometimes referred to as 'masked' allergies because, while their effects can be seen, the cause is unknown.

The only way to 'unmask' an allergy is, first, to withdraw the offending food and then, if the symptoms clear up, to confirm the diagnosis by reintroducing the food and seeing if the symptoms reappear.

The difficult question that your doctor or allergist may have to resolve is which foods to withdraw. If you invariably break out in a rash and start vomiting if you eat oysters, the diagnosis is pretty clear. But if your symptoms are more generalized and follow no clear pattern, or if they are delayed, the task can be very difficult. Specific food allergies are not inherited – only the tendency to become allergic – so there is little to be gained from a study of family history. Your medical consultant will probably need to make a thorough investigation of your lifestyle and personal history in order to gain clues as to what is wrong. Have you recently changed your diet – in order to slim, for example? Have you recently started using contraceptive pills? Are you taking sedatives or tranquillizers? Have you recently suffered from an infectious illness, such as hepatitis or 'flu? Are you exposed to other potential allergens at work or at home – an allergic response to your cat may be triggering your allergy to eggs, for example. An intolerance of alcohol is also often an indication of food allergy. All this information can provide valuable pointers as to whether you have a food allergy and, if so, what might be responsible.

You may also be given skin-prick or patch tests to identify the specific allergen. However, these are not particularly reliable in the case of food allergies and sometimes give false positive results.

ROTATION DIETS AND ELIMINATION DIETS

A rotation diet is one in which suspected foods are eaten and then avoided on a rotating basis. This might involve, for example, cutting out dairy products for three days out of four. A careful record should be kept. If the symptoms disappear for three days, and then recur on the fourth, you will have gone some way to identifying the problem.

An elimination diet (see p. 57) is designed both to eliminate symptoms and to aid identification of the cause. The diet will be based on your medical history and on any skin-prick or patch tests you have undergone, and it will be continued for several weeks. You may suffer withdrawal symptoms, such as headaches – a sure sign that you are allergic to the withdrawn food. Once the symptoms have completely disappeared, your doctor or allergist may reintroduce the foods one at a time, and watch for the reappearance of symptoms. This process is known as a 'challenge', and, in the case of children or particularly sensitive people, should be conducted only under medical supervision because of the danger of a severe anaphylactic reaction (see pp. 24–5).

In cases of mild food allergy, it is often possible for people to carry on eating the offending food occasionally and in small quantities. Food allergies can disappear for months or years before reappearing. If the reaction is severe, however, there is very little to be done. You will have no alternative but to resign yourself never to eat that particular food again, however tempting it may look!

MAIN CULPRITS

LIKELY CAUSES OF FOOD ALLERGY

Some food seem more likely than others to cause allergic reactions. Common culprits include:

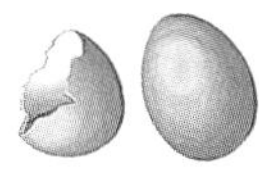
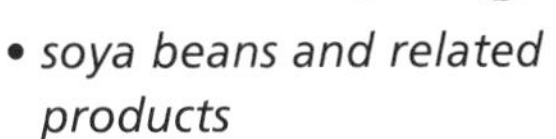
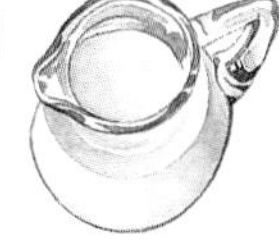

- *eggs*
- *milk*
- *soya beans and related products*
- *nuts (particularly peanuts)*
- *seafood (particularly shellfish)*
- *corn and wheat products*

Someone who is allergic to one particular type of food is often allergic to related foods. For example, an allergy to peanuts (which can cause very severe reactions) may mean an allergy to peas and beans and other members of the legume family.

Asthma

Many people don't think of asthma as an allergic disorder, and in a sense they are right. The fact is that asthma is really a set of symptoms that can be triggered by any of a number of factors – and allergens are among the most common of them. If it is severe, an attack of asthma can be life threatening, yet the sad fact is that the incidence of asthma is spiralling, in children in particular. Asthma is estimated to affect around 12.5 million people in the United States, for example, and in Britain alone it is known to kill around 2000 people a year. These statistics make asthma one of the most important of all allergic conditions.

A tendency towards asthma runs in families, just as a tendency to allergies does (see pp. 12–13), and children up to the age of about 17 are the most commonly affected. However, asthma can develop during adulthood, though it is thought that heredity has less of a part to play when this happens. The bronchioles, at the bottom of the lungs, are the smallest of the tubes that carry air. In an asthmatic they are sometimes described as 'twitchy' – that is, they narrow and tighten, as the muscles in the walls of the vessels contract.

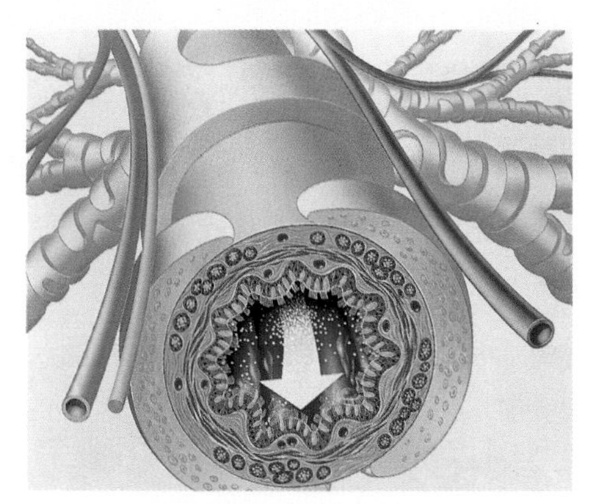

A bronchiole in section. Allergies can cause these tiny airways in the lung to tighten, triggering an asthmatic attack.

Triggered by any of a number of factors (see below), the involuntary contraction of the muscles narrows the airways; inflammation of the tissues further reduces the size of the airways; and mucous glands over-produce mucus, clogging up the airways. The result is that breathing becomes extremely difficult, and this can itself cause panic, so exacerbating the problem. The supply of oxygen to the tissues is reduced, and the results can be extremely serious.

ALLERGENS AND IRRITANTS

These effects are triggered by three types of factor: allergens, aspirin-containing products and irritants. Examples of allergens include pollen, flakes of animal skin, the droppings of house-dust mites, mould spores and certain foods. The distinction between allergens and the two other factors is important because neither aspirin nor irritants such as diesel fumes, smoke, perfume, paint and cold air (often a significant factor in asthma that is induced by exercise) cause an allergic reaction. They may stimulate receptors in the walls of the airways that make the muscle contract, but they do not cause histamine production (see pp. 10–11).

A CHRONIC PROBLEM

An attack of asthma can vary considerably both in its degree of severity and the length of time it lasts, from a few hours to several days. Unfortunately, the condition is chronic: – that is, persistent – and even though there may be intervals between attacks, and asthma may become less severe as you grow older, the potential that you will have an attack is always there.

Since an asthma attack is potentially so serious and there is always the risk that someone who has only previously had minor attacks may have a serious one, it should be stressed that natural remedies should not be used as an alternative to prescribed medical treatment during an asthma attack. To do so could be life-threatening. Breathing techniques, however, can be extremely useful when it comes to limiting the effects of an attack (see p. 21).

Natural remedies and common-sense avoidance measures do have the potential to help prevent an attack, however, and this is important, since the drugs used to treat asthma have various potential side-effects (see pp. 16–21). In particular, bronchodilators can, in some rare circumstances, cause an allergic response that actually triggers an attack.

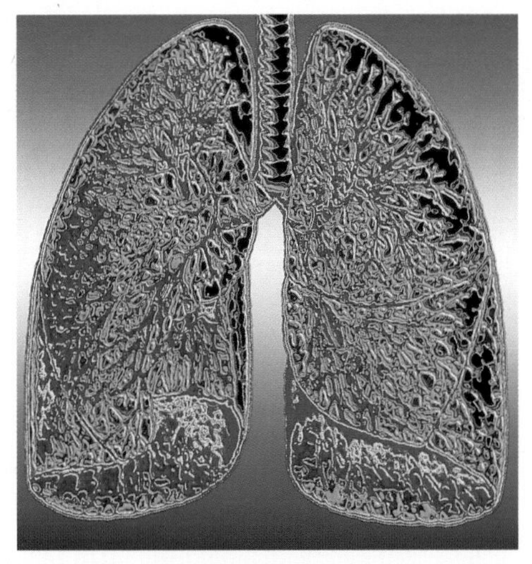

This computer-generated graphic shows the complex airways of the human lungs. The bronchioles are at the base.

BODY AND MIND

The reasons avoidance measures and preventive strategies (see pp. 102–23) are important are obvious, but it may be less evident why natural remedies should be effective. But it has been shown by experiment, time and time again, that stress and psychological factors play an important part in triggering an asthma attack – or, rather, in determining whether an asthma attack develops after exposure to a specific allergen. For example, in one experiment – which sounds rather unkind – a researcher released a small amount of pollen into the air when talking to a subject, without the subject knowing. When the pair were talking about non-controversial topics, the pollen had no effect, but when the conversation moved onto problems in the subject's emotional life, wheezing and breathing difficulties developed. This stopped when the subject was

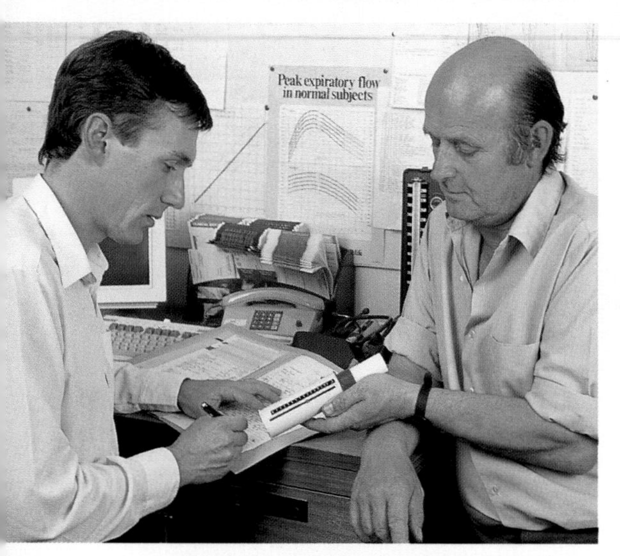

A doctor notes the reading on a peak-flow meter (see box below), used to measure lung capacity.

changed. Again, while we know that it is not true that children 'grow out of' asthma, since tests generally still show that the potential for an attack is present in later life, it is clear that adults suffer less from asthma because they have learned to cope with it and can avoid an attack because they have greater control of their emotions.

There is a good reason why this should be so. The smooth muscles in the wall of the bronchioles work without our conscious intervention. Along with other body systems, they are run automatically by the autonomic nervous system (see pp. 12–13). However, they still react to the presence of stress hormones, contracting

TESTS AND CURES

Conventional medicine also stresses the importance of relaxation and breathing techniques to asthmatics. However, one of the most useful tools in monitoring asthma – and, to a certain extent, in treating it – is the peak-flow meter. This measures something called the peak expiratory flow (PEF), which is just a way of saying how open your airways are. It is a simple device: you blow into it, and an indicator shows how much air can be blown out of your lungs – the more open the airways are, the more air you can blow. The significance of the PEF is that regular monitoring can indicate whether an attack is likely, because it will drop a few days before an attack develops.

Many asthmatics use peak-flow meters every day, keeping a chart or graph of their results, so that they can take preventive measures or medication (see pp. 16–21) to ward off an attack. Some types of peak-flow meters, used especially for children, have something called a 'windmill trainer' attached to them. This has sails that can be turned by the expiration of air, but it becomes more difficult to turn them the further up the scale it is fixed – this gives children something to aim at and improves their breathing techniques.

As yet, conventional medicine does not offer a cure for asthma, though research continues. Drugs that can help prevent an attack are available (see pp. 16–21), but during an attack there is only one medical response: first,to inhale bronchodilators , and, second, to use breathing and relaxation techniques. In the absence of any new 'wonder drug' to treat asthma, it remains important for asthmatics keep their inhalers nearby at all times.

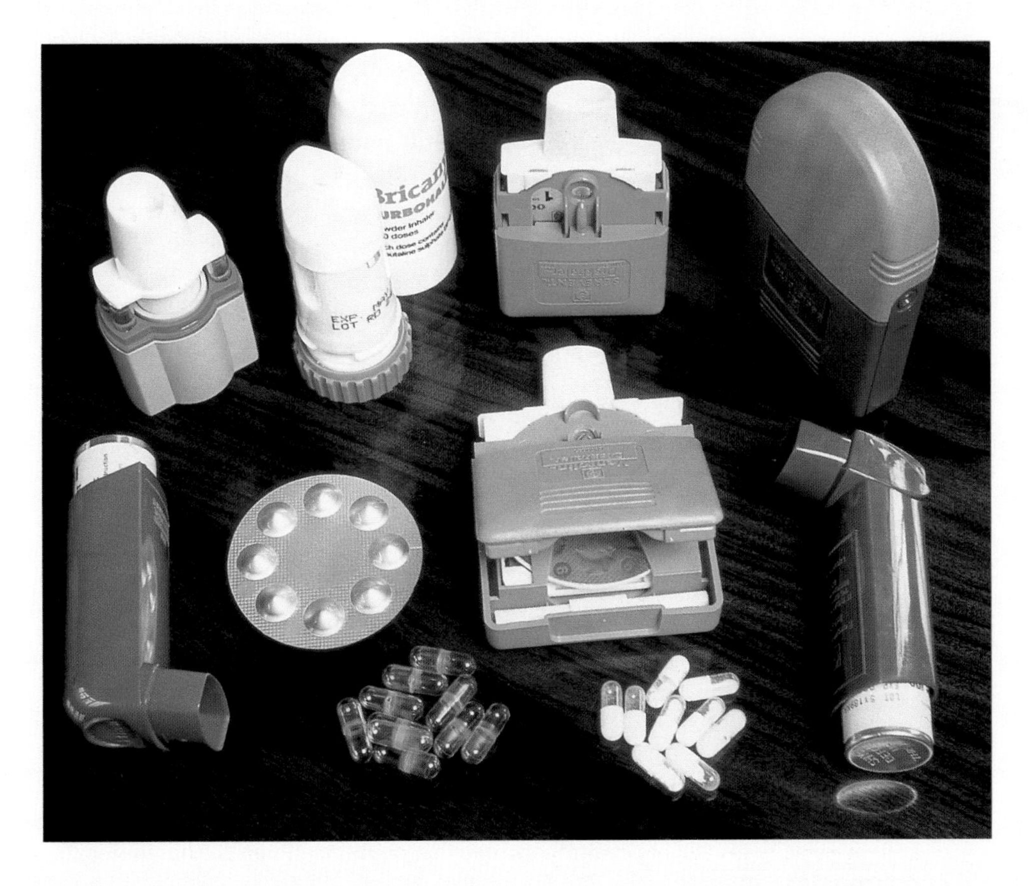

A selection of asthma inhalers and capsules, designed to deliver powerful drugs which either open airways in the lungs or reduce inflammation there. Relaxation and breathing exercises can offer an effective alternative to drugs, providing the sufferer with a greater sense of control over potential attacks.

and relaxing as appropriate. But as a child grows, he or she comes to learn that a certain amount of the functions of the autonomic nervous system can be influenced by the conscious mind. Some Indian holy men, for example, can lie on a bed of nails without experiencing pain. On a more mundane level, patients with high blood pressure can be taught to lower their pulse rate by breathing and relaxation techniques.

THE NATURAL WAY

What this means is that the natural strategies that are described in section three of this book play an important part in the prevention and control of asthma. They are: relaxation (see pp. 88–9); meditation (see pp. 96–7); visualization (see pp. 92–3); and yoga (see pp. 96–7). Use these together with the breathing exercises described earlier (see p. 21) and the methods taught by the Alexander Technique (see pp. 98–9), and you will have a whole range of natural weapons to use in the fight against asthma.

Ear and eye allergies

Anything that threatens the eyes or ears should be taken seriously. Fortunately, there are few allergic conditions that affect the ear. The eye is more vulnerable, but even here, few of the allergic conditions affecting the eye present a long-term threat to sight. Nevertheless, the eyes and ears are precious. If you suffer from repeated or persistent bouts of earache or of sore, reddened eyes, you should always consult your doctor.

EAR ALLERGIES

If you experience an itching sensation in the ear, together with a feeling that sounds are muffled and distorted, you may be suffering from an allergic reaction involving the middle ear. The condition is a form of otitis media, a common cause of earache, especially in children, which is usually caused by infection. However, otitis media is occasionally brought on by an allergy, and in this case it is nearly always linked to an attack of hayfever.

The problem is caused by blockage of the eustachian tube, the passage that links the back of the nasal passages to the middle ear. If the nasal membranes swell up badly as a result of an allergic reaction – to pollen grains, for example – they can block off the opening of the eustachian tube. When this happens, fluid from the middle ear is unable to drain away, so it accumulates and puts pressure on the eardrum. The fluid makes hearing difficult, and sometimes allows infection to develop.

TESTS AND CURES FOR EAR ALLERGIES

A doctor can easily check for fluid accumulation behind the eardrum using

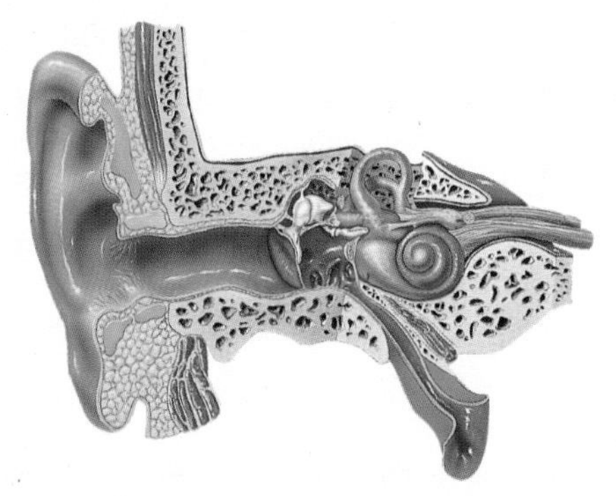

The middle ear is connected with the nasal passage and may become infected as a result of severe hayfever.

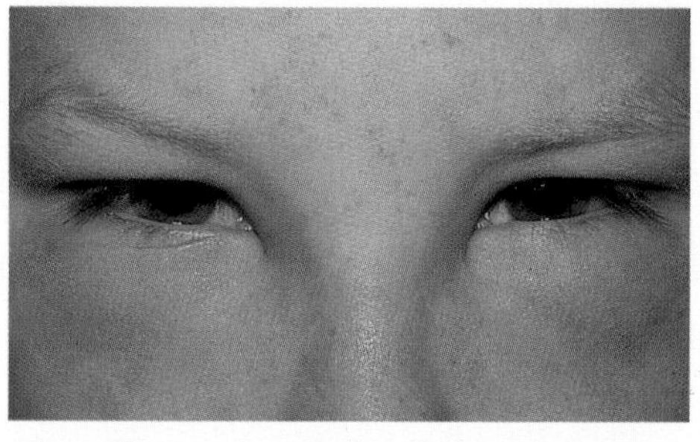

The effects of a pollen-induced reaction on the eyes. As well as puffiness and swelling, this patient is suffering from allergic conjunctivitis, whereby the eyes typically become red, watery and sore.

an otoscope. Children with suspected hearing difficulty might also be assessed with audiometry tests, which provide very accurate information about the child's ability to hear different types of sound at different levels of pitch and loudness. Usually, treatment with antihistamines or decongestants will reduce the swelling in the nose, unblocking the eustachian tube and allowing the middle ear to drain again. If the fluid accumulation persists, the ear may have to be drained using a simple procedure called a myringotomy.

Ear allergies are most likely to cause problems in childhood, at the time when a child is learning to talk. If the effect on hearing is not noticed and the condition is allowed to persist, the child may develop speech difficulties, and his or her education will suffer later on.

EYE ALLERGIES

Sore, red, itching and watering eyes are often linked to hayfever, and the cause is the same – an allergic response to pollen grains or some other allergen. The condition affects the conjunctiva, the white part of the eye, and is known as allergic conjunctivitis. It can affect one or both eyes. Sometimes the conjunctiva swells up, and the eye can become painfully sensitive to bright light.

Allergic conjunctivitis is usually an acute condition – that is, the symptoms appear rapidly, can be quite severe and normally disappear when the offending allergen is removed. In some cases, however, the acute condition can become long-lasting (or chronic). The eyes are likely to become dry and itchy, and vision may be blurred.

A rarer form of allergic conjunctivitis, known as vernal conjunctivitis, affects its victims (most often children) only in spring and summer. It causes the development of small hard bumps on the inner surface of the upper eyelids.

The eyes can also be affected by contact dermatitis (see pp. 48–9). In this case, the eyelids rather than the conjunctiva are affected, becoming thickened, cracked and dry. Very rarely, the cornea at the front of the eye is affected. If this happens, consult a doctor or ophthalmologist immediately.

TESTS AND CURES FOR EYE ALLERGIES

If the cause of your allergy is not already known, you may need to undergo standard skin prick or patch tests (see pp. 104–5) to identify the allergen responsible. Allergic conjunctivitis is usually treated with eye drops containing antihistamine and a vasoconstrictor (which narrows the blood vessels). Antihistamine is also often given orally. Severe cases can be treated with preparations containing steroids, which are also effective against vernal conjunctivitis and contact dermatitis. (Steroids should be used only under strict medical supervision, especially for eye conditions.) Finally, medications containing a form of sodium cromoglycate can be effective if used before symptoms appear, since they actually prevent the development of the allergic reaction.

Hayfever

Until this century, hayfever was a very rare condition – in fact, it was not identified as a medical disorder at all until 1819, and it was discovered that its cause is an allergy to pollen only in the 1870s. But since then, hayfever has become more and more common, to the point at which it is estimated that as many as one in six teenagers are affected by it. Typically, a hayfever sufferer has other family members who suffer from an allergy, though not necessarily hayfever, and first experiences symptoms during the teenage years, though later onset is not uncommon. Also, some 50 per cent of those who suffer from eczema during childhood develop hayfever later in life.

Strictly speaking, hayfever is known medically as seasonal allergic rhinitis , which is caused only by an allergy pollen of a particular type. The pollens involved are most often those from plants in which pollen is wind-borne; plants that are pollinated by insects, such as most cultivated flowers, rarely cause hayfever. However, the term is also generally used to describe an allergic reaction to other allergens that are often present all year round, such as the droppings of house-dust mites, or animal proteins – from cats and dogs and so on. Medically, this condition is referred to as perennial allergic rhinitis. The difference between the two is further confused by the phenomenon of cross-reactions (see pp. 14–15), which means that someone who is allergic to pollen can experience

HAYFEVER AND ASTHMA

A minority of hayfever sufferers also suffer from 'pollen asthma', a form of asthma triggered in the main by pollen, although other allergens that cause allergic rhinitis can also be responsible. The mechanism that causes the problem is not entirely clear. It may be that tiny fragments of the allergens reach the lungs by being inhaled or, as some scientists believe, it may be that an attack of hayfever makes the bronchi (the tubes that carry air to the base of the lungs) hypersensitive to other asthma triggers, such as cold air or diesel fumes.

Whatever the case, an asthma attack is potentially a very serious event (see pp. 34–7). Generally, the asthmatic attacks associated with pollen asthma are not particularly significant, and the symptoms pass quickly – they can be overcome, too, by the use of breathing techniques (see pp. 20 – 21). However, if you have hayfever and you suffer from wheeziness, a tight chest and a dry cough from time to time, you should consult your doctor, because such attacks can sometimes become considerably worse and it may be wise to have medication on hand.

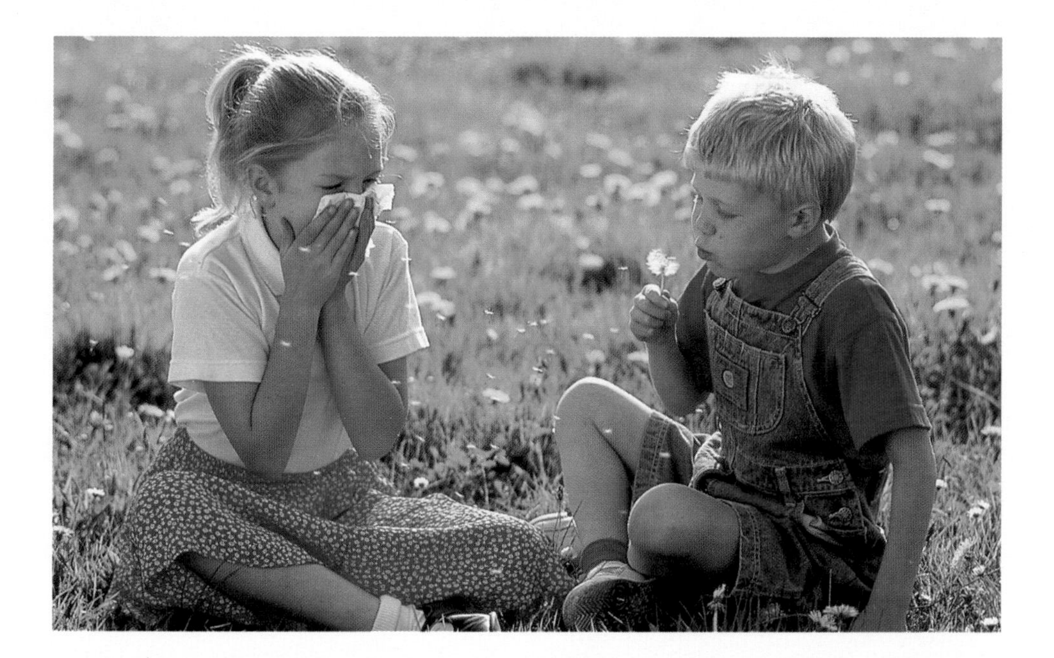

Pollen from grass and wildflowers is a common cause of hayfever's typical sneezes and snuffles.

symptoms when exposed to house-dust mite droppings, for example.

GAUGING A PASSAGEWAY

In both types of allergic rhinitis the mechanism is essentially the same: tiny particles of the allergen are breathed in and antibodies respond to the presence of foreign proteins by attracting mast cells, which in turn produce histamine (see pp. 10–11). However, what makes the symptoms of true pollen hayfever so much more severe than other types is one particular quality of the pollen. The purpose of a grain of pollen is to pollinate another plant and reproduce the species, but in order to do this it has to force its way through the stigma of a flower to reach the egg cell within it. To do this, the pollen first releases proteins that identify it as being of the correct species and then releases protein enzymes that gauge a passageway through the stigma. When a grain of pollen meets the lining of a human nose, it reacts in exactly the same way: first, identifying proteins are released, and then protein enzymes follow. The body responds to this attempted invasion of proteins vigorously, and the allergic response starts.

THE SYMPTOMS

The first sign of an attack is a tingling, itchy feeling in the eyes, nose, mouth and throat, which indicates that the body has begun to react to the presence of an allergen. In the second stage, which follows fairly quickly, the body tries to expel the foreign particles physically: the nose and eyes start to run, to flush out the particles; then a succession of sneezes attempts to expel them more forcibly. Unfortunately, the

TESTS AND CURES

In the case of hayfever, it is particularly useful to know your enemy, because you can then take special precautions (see pp. 100–23) during the time of year when the pollen to which you are allergic has its season. You can also avoid any plants from the same botanical family, and watch out for any known cross-reactions. There are a variety of ways of discovering the precise type of pollen or other allergen to which you are allergic – skin tests, patch tests and provocative testing (see pp. 104–105) – but they work on the same general principle: a variety of suspected allergens are introduced to the body and the sites observed to see which one becomes inflamed. The process is simple but effective.

Identification is one thing, cure is another. Desensitization therapy is sometimes effective, but it takes a long time, is available only in special clinics and can be dangerous (see pp. 16–21). The symptoms of hayfever can be relieved by a range of drugs such as antihistamines, sympathomimetics, corticosteroids and mast cell stabilizers, but at the risk of various side-effects (see pp. 16–21).

sneeze reaction is something of a lost cause, because more particles are taken in with every breath.

While this first line of defence is being activated, antibodies are latching on to the allergens and marking them for the attention of the mast cells (see pp. 10–11). These flock to the site, releasing histamine to destroy the invaders, which, in turn, irritates and inflames the membranes, making them swell up. In the nose, this blocks the passageways, which are already having to cope with the copious quantities of mucus that are being produced; in the case of the eyes, this inflammation may involve the eyeball, giving rise to conjunctivitis (see pp. 38–39).

The third stage of an attack of hayfever – or of any type of allergic rhinitis – involves the spread of inflammation to other areas. The bones of the face and skull are not solid, but contain a honeycomb of cavities, called the sinuses, and mucus and, sometimes, foreign particles, can travel into them from the nose and mouth, especially when it is being produced in such quantities. This mucus may become infected, causing further inflammation, and the consequent increase in pressure often causes severe headaches in the forehead and aches and pains in the cheeks.

The inner ear often becomes involved in an attack of hayfever, too, because it is linked to the nasal cavity by means of the eustachian tube. Mucus can overflow into this tube, blocking it and giving an unpleasant sensation of tightness (see pp. 38–39)

The severity of all these symptoms depends on a variety of factors: how much of the allergen you are exposed to and for how long; how frequently exposure recurs; how quickly and effectively symptoms are treated; and the nature of your individual reaction, both in physiological and emotional terms.

Not only do hayfever symptoms persist, they can actually get worse day by day. The immune system continues to overreact, and re-exposure even to small quantities of an allergen intensifies the condition.

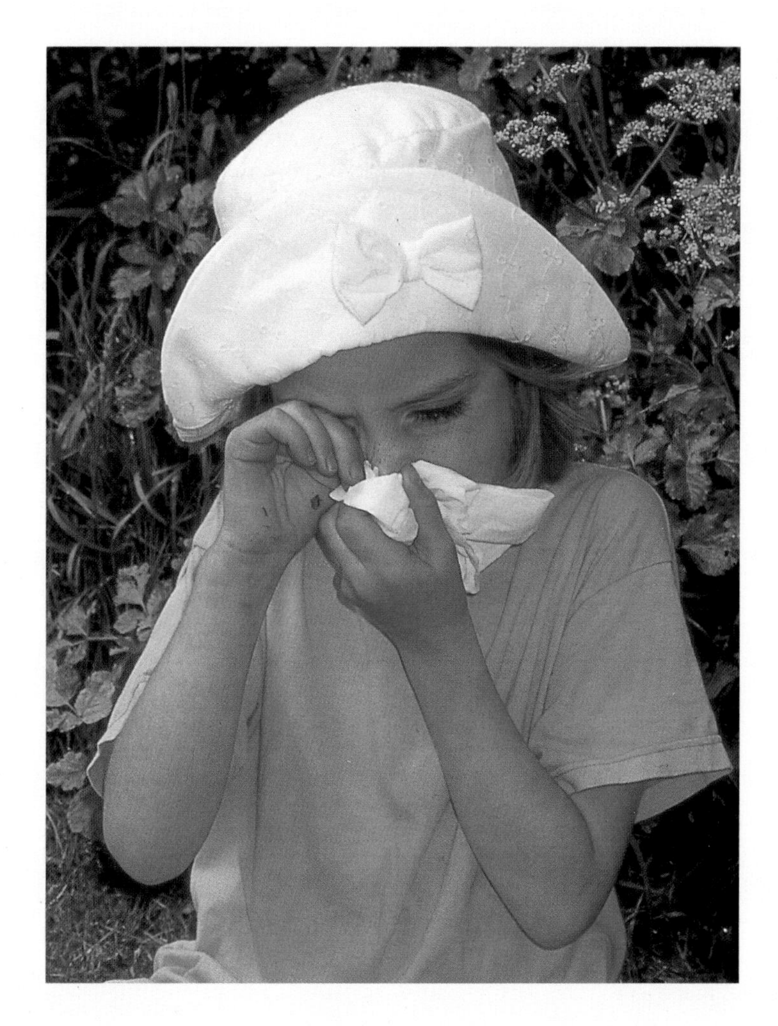

PRIMING AND LATE-PHASE REACTIONS

Hayfever differs from many other allergies in that its symptoms often become worse, day by day. There are two reasons for this. The first is a phenomenon known as 'priming'. By the nature of the problem, hayfever sufferers are repeatedly exposed to their allergen, and more antibodies are created on each exposure. This means that on every new exposure to pollen, more mast cells will be attracted to the site and more histamine will be produced – making the symptoms more intense.

The second reason is something called 'late-phase reaction'. This refers to the fact that some types of immune cells (the neutrophils and basophils) take longer to reach the site of an allergen than others (see p. 10). The result is that the nose of a hayfever sufferer may become inflamed once more many hours after the original attack has died down. This constant inflammation makes the membranes of the nose become increasingly sensitive – so that a smaller quantity of allergen will be sufficient to re-trigger the condition.

Hives

Hives, or urticaria, can be an extremely distressing condition. The skin can itch so intensely that sufferers may be unable to sleep or work. Fortunately, most cases are mild and short-lived. An example of hives with which most people are familiar is nettle rash. But even this mild form of hives can cause considerable discomfort for a few minutes or hours, as anyone unwary enough to have wandered into a bed of young nettles will be all too painfully aware. It is estimated that 20 per cent of the population will suffer from hives at some stage in their lives. Allergic individuals are more likely to suffer than others, but there are many causes of hives beside allergies, and non-allergic hives is common.

Hives begins with an itchy skin. Within a short period of time, a raised whitish or reddish lump – a hive – appears. Hives can take many different shapes and forms and can appear anywhere on the body, either as individual swellings in different parts of the body, or as clusters of small swellings concentrated in a particular area. Sometimes hives merge together, forming a large area of swelling. Each hive generally lasts less than a day, but further eruptions normally take place in another part of the body.

Hives is said to be acute if it lasts for less than six weeks, and chronic if it lasts for longer than six weeks. Most cases are acute – many last only for a few hours.

WHAT CAUSES HIVES?

There are literally thousands of possible causes of hives. Allergens can reach the body through contact with the skin, they can be injected, eaten or drunk, or, less often, they can be inhaled. Drugs are one of the commonest causes – penicillin and other antibiotics, aspirin and related anti-inflammatory drugs, sulfonamides and codeine are often culprits.

Food is another common cause. Dairy products, eggs, shellfish, peanuts and other nuts are all known to contain allergens that can trigger an attack of hives. Food additives can have the same effect – tartrazine dyes and preservatives such as sodium benzoate seem to be the worst offenders. Insect bites and stings can produce reactions ranging from a few localized hives to the dangerous generalized reaction known as anaphylactic shock (see pp. 24–5). Contact with latex can have the same result. Vaccinations can cause serum sickness (see pp. 28–29), which includes hives. Virus infections, such as glandular fever and infectious hepatitis, and bacterial infections, such as 'strep throat', are thought to be the triggers for some cases of hives, as are parasitic infestations.

There are also a number of physical causes of hives. Heat, cold, pressure on the skin, vibration, exposure to sunlight, exercise or stress may all bring about an attack. These are not allergies, although people often describe them as such.

WHAT HAPPENS IN AN ATTACK OF HIVES?

The underlying reaction in hives is the same as in other allergic conditions. The body's immune system overreacts to the presence of the allergen by producing histamine (see pp. 10–11). When this happens in the skin, the small blood vessels under the skin's surface begin to leak fluid into the surrounding tissue. The fluid irritates the nerve endings, which also lie just under the surface, causing itching and discomfort. The fluid also produces the swellings or hives.

ANGIODERMA

This allergic reaction is similar to hives but involves tissues lying deeper under the skin. The areas of swelling tend to be larger than in hives, but there is seldom any itching because the nerve endings concerned don't occur at these deeper levels. Angioedema can, however, cause pain if the swelling is so large that it puts pressure on surrounding tissues, or if it stretches the skin in areas where it is tight. Swelling most often affects the lips, eyelids, hands and feet.

Unlike hives, angioedema can, in certain circumstances, be life-threatening. If it affects the mouth or tongue, or the throat, the swelling can severely restrict breathing. Immediate medical attention is required in order to establish an airway and ensure that the body receives an adequate supply of oxygen.

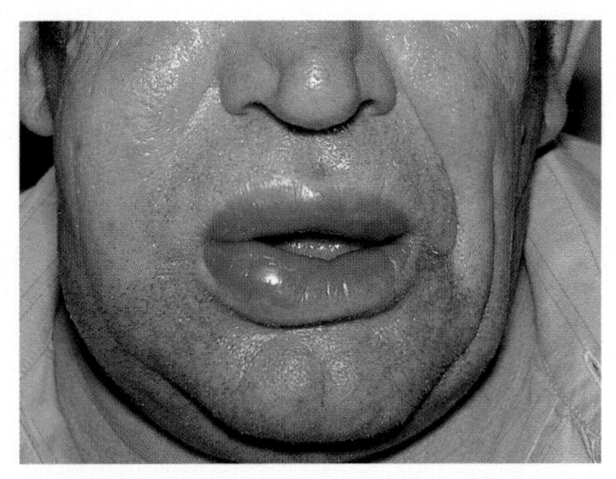

Angioderma, seen here as a swelling of the mouth and lips, is a hives-like allergic reaction in deeper tissues.

TESTS AND CURES

Hives and angioedema are relatively easy to identify from the symptoms, supported by blood and urine tests. It can be much more difficult to identify the cause – in fact, the cause remains unknown in a majority of cases. If your hives is thought to be the result of an allergy, the same techniques that are used in other forms of allergy (see pp. 104–105) can be used to try to identify the allergen responsible.

Hives is nearly always treated with antihistamines, and normally no other treatment is required. However, a severe outbreak of hives or angioedema may need injections of adrenaline as an emergency measure. Steroids are almost always effective but, because of their undesirable side-effects, these powerful drugs would normally be used only if treatment with antihistamines fails, and must be taken under proper supervision from your doctor.

Insect stings

Insect stings have been one of the banes of the human race throughout history. Occasionally they cause death. The first written record of a fatal sting takes the form of a hieroglyphic account of the death after being stung by a wasp of the Egyptian Pharaoh Menes in 2641 BC . Today, millions of people are stung by insects every year, but very few suffer anything more than a short period of discomfort. Only about one person in 200 will suffer more serious symptoms, usually due to an allergy, and only a small fraction of these will die of an acute and severe allergic response.

The culprit in almost all stinging attacks belongs to an order of insects known as Hymenoptera. This group includes bees (including the honeybee and the bumble bee), wasps and hornets. In North America, fire ants and yellow jackets are a source of trouble. There are occasionally reports of an influx of dangerous insects from Europe or Africa, for example, usually called 'killer bees'. The reports are often exaggerated and the insects concerned are normally no more poisonous than the home-grown varieties, although they may be more aggressive.

Only female insects sting. In honeybees, the sting is attached to the gut and the sting itself is barbed. When the bee tries to extract the sting, it loses much of its insides and dies. As a result, honeybees are mainly unaggressive and tend to sting only to protect the hive or when stepped on. Bumblebees are also peaceful and need a lot of provocation before they will sting. Wasps and hornets, on the other hand, are much more easily annoyed and can deliver a painful sting. Hornets particularly are notoriously bad tempered, and deliver a vicious sting. Keep out of their way.

REACTIONS TO INSECT STINGS

Stinging insects produce a poisonous venom, which they inject into the skin. In most cases, the pain, local inflammation and swelling are due to the toxic effects of the venom on the tissues surrounding the site of the sting. Only seldom do the toxic effects spread to other parts of the body. When they do, it is invariably the result of a large number of stings over a short period of time, introducing such large quantities of venom that it has spread around the body.

Except in the case of multiple stings, any reaction that involves parts of the body at a distance from the site of the sting is a certain indication that an allergic reaction is taking place. If hives, gross swelling or breathing difficulties occur, then it is likely that a generalized allergic response known as anaphylactic shock (see pp. 24–5) is taking place, and immediate medical attention is required. An allergic reaction to an insect sting can occur only once an individual has been

Bees sting only in extreme circumstances as the sting is fatal to the bee. Wasps and hornets sting at will. Skin tests with specific insect venoms can reveal potential sensitivity to insect stings.

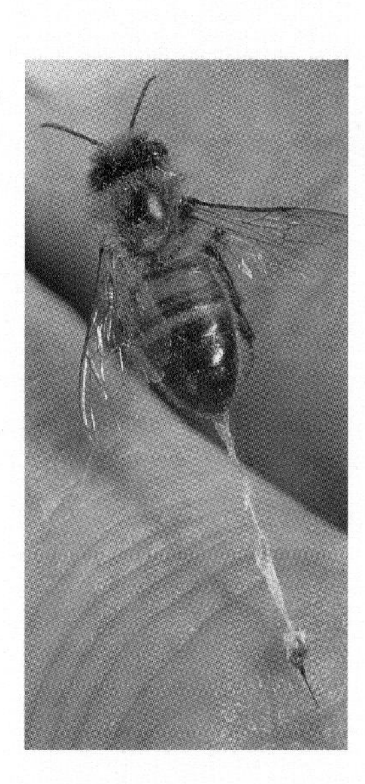

sensitized – that is, after already having been stung. On the first occasion, the response is likely to be similar to a non-allergic reaction. The next time the individual is stung, the full allergic response comes into play.

TESTS AND CURES

People who react badly to insect stings should be tested for an allergy because of the risk of anaphylactic shock in any subsequent attack. Skin tests, using specific insect venoms, are accurate; blood tests are less so.

Once the allergy has been confirmed, there are various precautions that can be taken, of which avoidance is obviously the first (see box). The second is to carry a loaded syringe of adrenaline, which your doctor can prescribe. Finally, desensitization therapy should be considered (see pp. 18–19), especially if planning to visit high-risk areas. Because of the severity of anaphylactic shock, desensitization can be life-saving.

AVOIDING INSECT STINGS

If you are allergic to insect stings, there are some measures that you should take to avoid being stung.

- *Cover up well; don't go barefoot or wear shorts or short sleeves when out of doors, particularly in grassy areas or places where insects feed.*
- *Wear gloves while gardening.*
- *Avoid cosmetics, hair sprays, deodorants and perfumes, all of which can attract insects.*
- *Be careful when cooking and eating out of doors.*
- *Avoid brightly coloured clothes, particularly floral prints, as these are very attractive to insects.*
- *Keep a can of insecticide spray at home and in the car.*
- *Keep your emergency adrenaline injection kit close to hand at all times.*
- *Wear a tag or bracelet stating what your condition is; if you collapse, this will help to make sure that you get the correct treatment promptly.*

OTHER INSECT ALLERGIES

Almost everyone is familiar with the swelling and irritation produced by mosquitoes and some types of flies. These are bites, not stings, and the reaction is not allergic. Very rarely, there have been cases of severe allergic response to bedbugs, and some caterpillars (notably those of the brown-tail and yellow-tail moths) are well known to produce an allergic response, although this is usually mild. In general, the best way to deal with these allergies is to avoid the cause.

Skin allergies

Skin is one of the most sensitive, as well as the most public, of all the body's tissues. It is also in constant contact with the outside world. The general term for skin inflammation, often allied with rashes of raised spots or scales, is eczema, and allergic eczema is very common. It is an uncomfortable and often embarrassing condition. Children with bad eczema may become withdrawn and unsociable, and their performance at school may deteriorate. Adults may have to change jobs if their work brings them in contact with substances to which they are allergic.

Patches of red, itchy skin are the main feature of eczema. The skin becomes dry. Blisters may develop – often as a result of scratching – and the skin may break and take on a watery, 'weeping' appearance. These areas are fertile breeding grounds for bacteria, and infection is common. In long-term eczema, the skin becomes thicker, leathery and dark. There are two main types of allergic eczema. The first is known as contact eczema, or contact dermatitis, because it involves direct skin contact. The second is known as atopic eczema, and occurs in people who are atopic – that is, they are particularly susceptible to allergies (see pp. 12–13).

CONTACT ECZEMA

Many people experience a mild, but irritating, reaction to metals such as nickel, and may not be able to wear a particular necklace or a watch with a metal back. Other common causes of

COPING WITH EZCEMA

A few simple precautions can reduce the severity of eczema and give welcome relief from constant itching.

- *Use moisturizers regularly to counteract dry skin; add moisturizing oils to your bath.*
- *Avoid soaps and detergents; hypoallergenic preparations are available from chemists.*
- *Wear rubber gloves when doing household chores involving water or detergents.*
- *Wear cotton clothing rather than wool; wool next the skin makes itching worse.*
- *Keep children's nails short and smooth; put cotton mittens on their hands at night to prevent scratching.*
- *Maintain an even temperature in your home – around 68°–70°F (20°–22°C); your itching gets worse if you get too hot and start sweating.*
- *Use a humidifier if the air in your home is dry.*

allergic contact eczema include drugs, soaps, bleaches, detergents, hair-dyes, nail-varnish and lipstick. Some plant substances, particularly primulas and chrysanthemums, can produce a reaction, The list of potential allergens is very long and would include most of the materials and chemicals used in the modern world. The rash caused by contact eczema is usually confined to the area of contact. However, repeated exposure may cause the rash to spread. Avoidance of the allergen will cure the condition, but this may be difficult if your occupation involves daily contact with it. Ultimately, people with sensitivity to allergens in the workplace may have to change their jobs.

ATOPIC ECZEMA

This type of eczema is strongly associated with a family history of allergy. It can appear at an early age – usually before the age of one, when it is termed infantile eczema, and can be very distressing. The rash, accompanied by severe itching, usually appears first on the cheeks, later spreading to the neck, scalp, the backs of the ears, the arms and the sides of the legs. If the condition continues or recurs, the skin becomes very dry, and develops a leathery texture from constant scratching. The rash tends to be confined to the face, the neck, the elbow creases, and behind the knees.

Food can trigger atopic eczema, and in cases involving babies milk is often the chief suspect. House-dust mites may be another cause. Most cases of infantile eczema – about 85 per cent – clear up spontaneously during childhood.

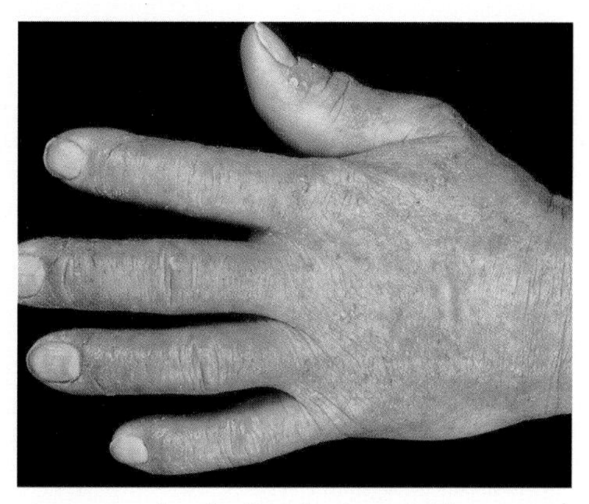

An example of allergic dermatitis, caused in this case by contact with cement.

TESTS AND CURES

The treatment of eczema tends to rely mainly on controlling the inflammation and itching, and, if it can be identified, avoiding the allergen concerned. Skin prick or patch tests (see pp. 104–105) can be used in the case of contact eczema. For atopic eczema, an elimination diet (see pp. 32–33) is the usual test.

The most effective way of reducing itching is to use antihistamines. Different antihistamines may need to be tried before the most effective one is found. Steroid creams and ointments help reduce inflammation but require medical supervision in their use because of possible side-effects. Cold water or aluminium acetate solution compresses can be useful for alleviating the itching and inflammation of a severe outbreak. For long-term eczema, tar preparations are sometimes recommended to control inflammation and itching. In addition to these medical treatments, there is much that you can do yourself to reduce the discomfort and severity of eczema (see p. 48).

Total allergy syndrome

Open your newspaper in the morning, and there's a good chance that you'll see a headline: 'Ten-year-old boy allergic to life'. And since the phrase was first coined, about 15 years ago, there have been numerous reports of people who, it is claimed, suffer from 'total allergy syndrome'. But does the condition really exist? As you would expect where allergies are concerned, the answer is far from clear cut.

When you see a picture of a child inside a polythene tent and read a claim that he or she is 'allergic to life', you can be fairly certain that the journalist responsible is misusing the word 'allergy'. Such children suffer from conditions in which their immune systems do not function adequately – unless they were protected from the outside world, they would be exposed to infections against which they have no defences and that would almost certainly be fatal. This is the direct opposite of an allergy, in which the immune system, and in particular the aggressive mast cell response (see pp. 10–11), responds too efficiently against something that is an inappropriate target. The condition is caused by a faulty gene, and in some instances has been cured by gene therapy, in which a healthy gene is introduced into the patient's body.

NO NORMAL LIFE

The newspaper reports are not always wrong, however. On rare occasions, doctors and researchers come across people who have such a range of severe allergies that they are sometimes said to be suffering from 'total allergy syndrome', mainly because nobody knows how else to characterize their condition. In such cases, normal life is nearly impossible. Sufferers find that all their time is spent trying to avoid potential allergens, undergoing desensitization therapy (see pp. 16–21) wearing industrial masks and living on almost perpetual exclusion diets which are themselves unhealthy and potentially dangerous. To make matters worse, long-term use of the types of drug that can be used to control allergic symptoms is dangerous – especially in the case of steroids (see pp. 16–21).

But the question is: why do some people suffer from a wide range of allergies? Opinions vary. Some doctors believe that other conditions, such as depressive illnesses or myalgic encephalopathy (ME), are responsible; other authorities take the view that poisoning by organophosphates or some other chemical is the cause.

There is certainly some evidence to support the latter view. One 16-year-old girl who has had to live with total allergy syndrome since she was a baby was recently found to have unusually high levels of tin in her blood. Tin is know to be highly toxic, and it is also known that tin persists in the body for an extraordinarily long time. When she was a baby, her garden was next to a field in which potatoes were grown, and at that time potatoes were often sprayed with a fungicide that contained organo-tin compounds. And the final piece of the jigsaw is that all her hair fell out many years ago – and Cornish tin miners were once notorious for their lack of hair.

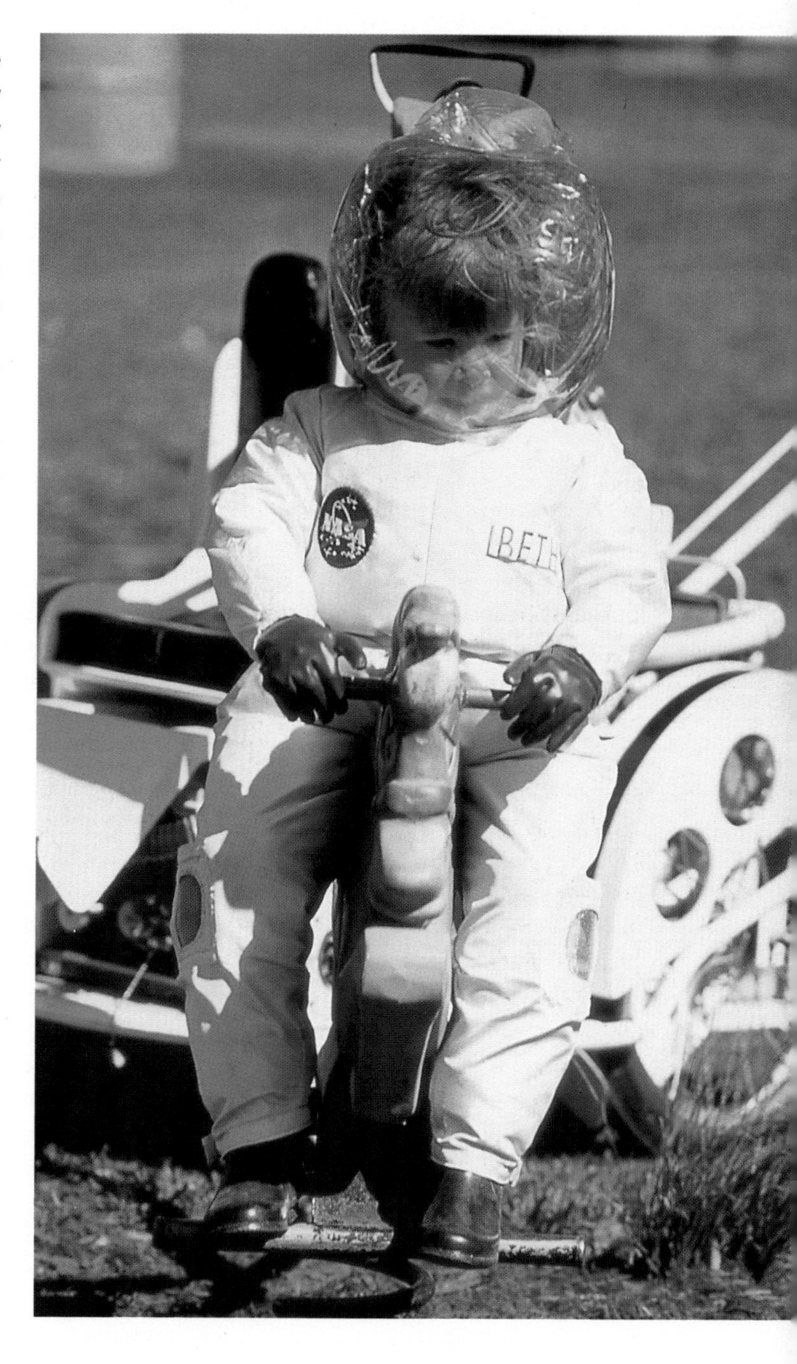

This biological isolation garment is the only device capable of screening out all potential allergens, but is practical for only comparatively short periods of time.

As yet, nobody knows why poisoning with tin or organophosphates should cause total allergy syndrome – if, indeed, they do. However, it is not impossible that ongoing research will come up with an answer to the problem, especially because so-called 'Gulf War Syndrome', which also involves allergies in some cases and is believed by many to be the result of organophosphate poisoning, is the subject of a good deal of research in Britain and the United States.

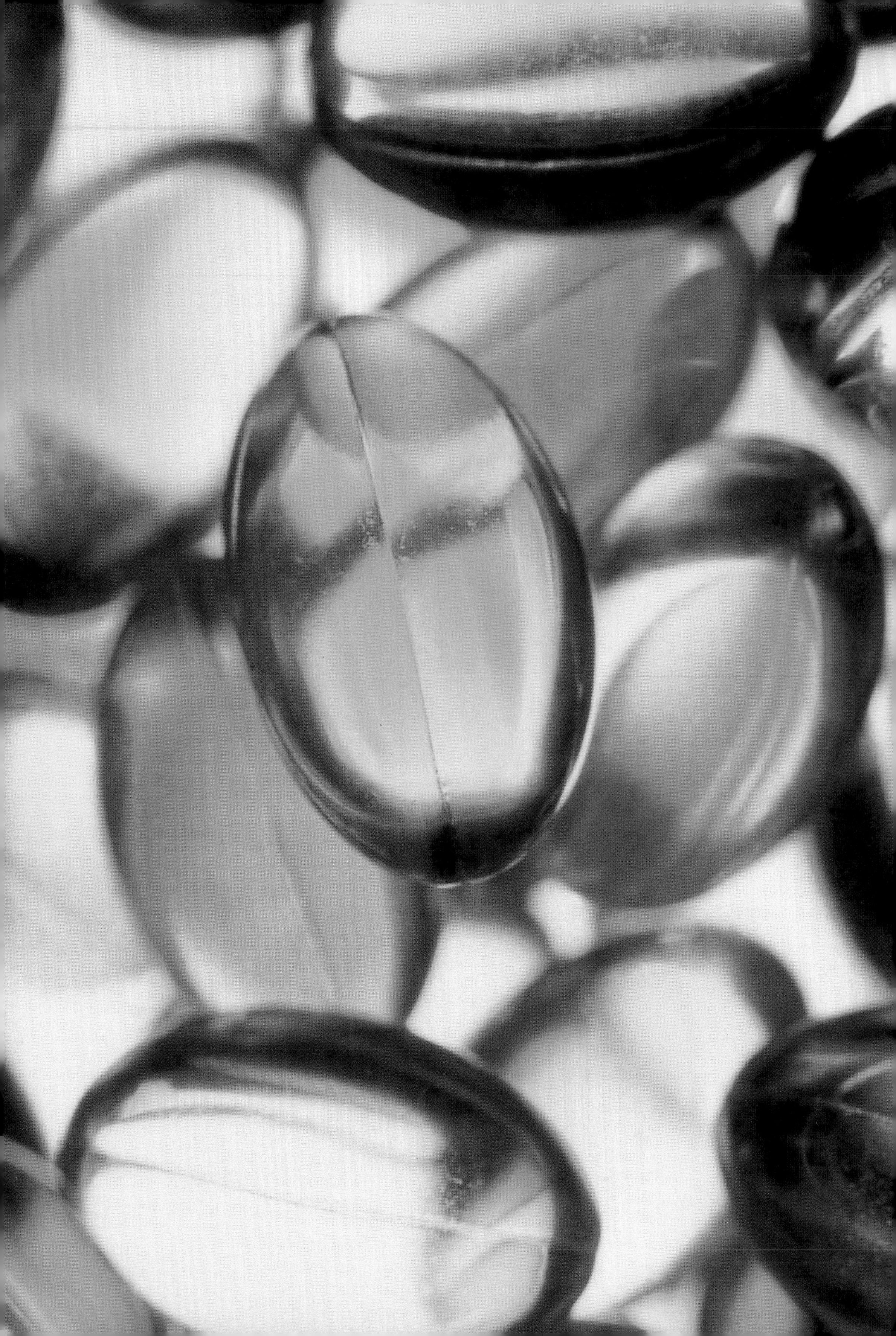

CHAPTER 3

Natural remedies and alternative treatments

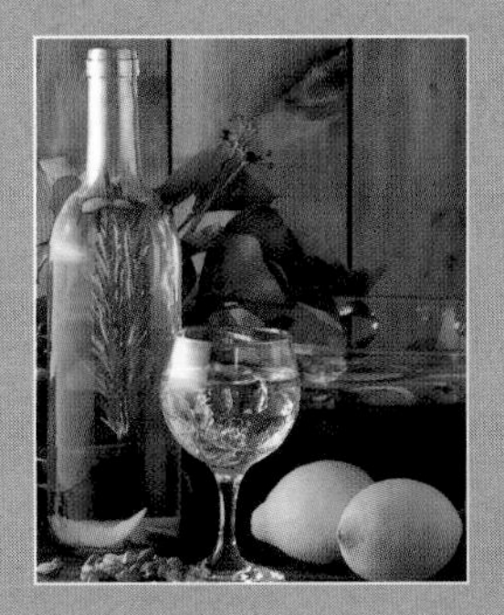

Now that you know how allergies work and the symptoms that they produce, it is easier to see what can be done to treat them, both preventively and when an allergic reaction occurs. This section of the book shows how the body's natural healing abilities can be harnessed effectively to help reduce the misery that allergies can cause. However, allergies can be serious and life-threatening, so the measures recommended here should not be used as an alternative to taking any prescribed medication or to seeking immediate medical advice in the acute stage of any allergic response.

DIET AND NUTRITION • NATUROPATHY HERBAL REMEDIES • HOMEOPATHY • FLOWER REMEDIES • ACUPUNCTURE • ACUPRESSURE REFLEXOLOGY • MASSAGE AND AROMATHERAPY RELAXATION AND EXERCISE • HYPNOTHERAPY VISUALIZATION • MEDITATION AND YOGA ALEXANDER TECHNIQUE

Diet and nutrition

Many people believe that one reason why the incidence of allergies has increased is that our immune system no longer develops properly. As a result of this, the body does not possess sufficient numbers of the antibodies that can attract cells that work gently, over a period (see pp. 10–11), to destroy antigens, and so help is needed from the more aggressive mast cells, which cause many of the symptoms of an allergic reaction. One culprit for this lack of development is thought to be our dependence on refined foods. So dietary and nutritional measures can help the immune system to develop properly and boost the level of the antibodies that help destroy allergens without giving rise to symptoms, and may also help reduce their severity.

FOODS TO AVOID

Here is a list of foods to avoid, because they depress the immune system, increase the chances that an allergic response will occur or will make the symptoms of one worse

A selection of healthy foods. Pulses such as chickpeas, lentils and beans (in the bowls) contain essential B vitamins.

Dairy products Reduce the amount of dairy products you consume, milk in particular, during the spring and summer because they increase the body's ability to produce mucus and catarrh. This measure is recommended by Ayurvedic practitioners, who believe that many chronic diseases are worsened by an unbalanced diet and that an excess of dairy products creates an imbalance

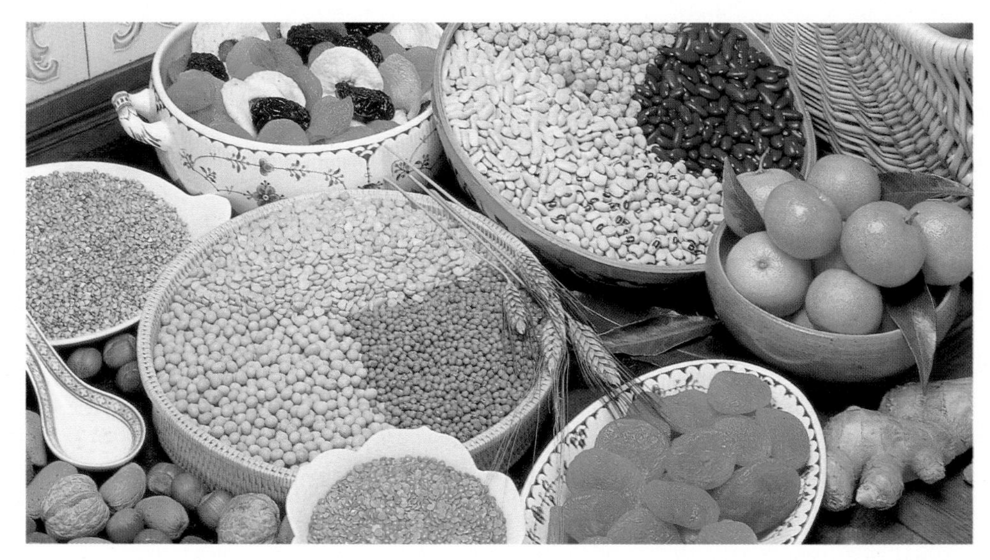

between the three basic forces that control the functioning of the body and maintain the 'prana', or life-force.

Sugar and wheat Grass pollens come from the same botanical family as sugar and wheat, so it is worthwhile cutting down on them in your diet if you suffer from hayfever.

Refined carbohydrates Research has shown that these depress the immune system within an hour of being eaten. White bread, sweets, cake and chocolate are all refined carbohydrates.

Animal fats The effects of animal fats on the immune system are not certain, but it is thought that a diet high in them can reduce the system's efficiency.

FOODS TO CHOOSE

Vitamins B5 (pantothenic acid), B6 and C are natural antihistamines, as are magnesium and folic acid. On the other hand, vitamins B, C and E, taken with a supply of protein, help promote a healthy immune system. A balanced diet should contain all these ingredients.

ZINC

This mineral is essential for the proper functioning of the immune system. It is contained in the following foods: crabmeat, oysters, white turkey meat, baked potato skins, shellfish, pulses, cottage cheese, bran, milk and red meats.

MEDICAL WATCHPOINT

If you are taking iron supplements – because you are pregnant, for example, or you have anaemia – you should not take zinc supplements or eat an excessive amount of foods that contain it unless asked to do so by your doctor: one affects the absorption of the other.

MAGNESIUM

A natural antihistamine, this mineral plays a vital role in many aspects of the body's chemistry, including the immune system. An increased intake of magnesium has been shown to reduce the frequency and severity of hayfever attacks. It can be found in the following foods: nuts, winkles, shrimps, soya beans and green leafy vegetables (the darker green the better).

VITAMIN B5

Also known as pantothenic acid, this vitamin is valuable in combating excess histamine. It is found in eggs, whole grain cereals and white meat.

IMMUNE SYSTEM SUPPRESSORS

There are many reasons why you should not smoke and why you should avoid alcohol, and caring for your immune system is one of them. Alcohol and smoking deplete the body's store of the B vitamins and zinc, both of which are vital if the immune system is to function properly. And alcohol's effect on the liver inhibits the production of a chemical that helps break down histamine, so if you drink alcohol your symptoms are likely to persist for longer.

MEDICAL WATCHPOINT

Consult your doctor before embarking on an elimination or exclusion diet.

VITAMIN B6

This vitamin is essential in the processing of several vital chemicals required by the immune system. It is contained in foods such as kidney beans, chicken, sunflower seeds, tuna, spinach, pulses and rice.

FOLIC ACID

Another member of the vitamin B group, folic acid is essential for the functioning of the central nervous system, and it is particularly important for health in the vulnerable years of early childhood. It can be found in a wide range of foodstuffs, including liver and kidneys, yeast, chickpeas, orange juice, soya beans and spinach, broccoli, cabbage, cauliflower beetroot, pulses, banana, and other fresh fruit and vegetables.

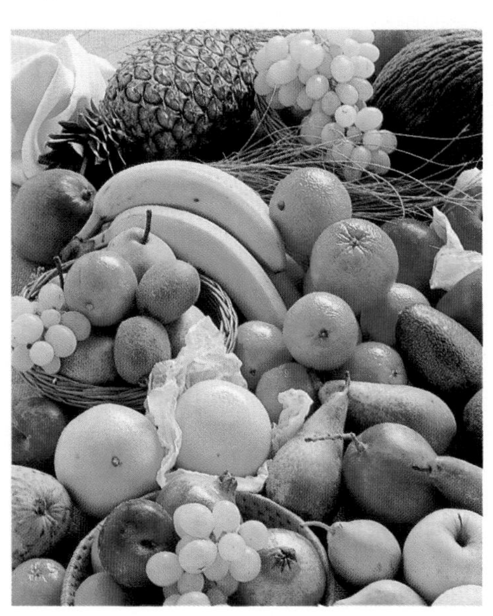

Over a few weeks, a food diary like this (opposite) can help reveal the nature of a food allergy. This one indicates a possible reaction to chocolate: both stomach pain and itchiness of the lips can be signs of an allergic response, albeit a mild one. But you should discuss the diary with your doctor before taking any action.

VITAMIN C

This vitamin is involved in very many chemical processes in the body. It is a powerful antioxidant – a group of chemicals that boosts the immune system – and helps in the production of important hormones. (Many claims have been made for vitamin C, including its effectiveness in curing cancer and the common cold, but not all doctors accept these. Nevertheless there appears to be no harm in maintaining a generous intake of the vitamin.) Vitamin C is found in foods such as broccoli, cabbage, citrus fruit, spinach, tomatoes, banana, carrots and all fruit and vegetables.

MEDICAL WATCHPOINT

Growing children need plenty of calcium to build their bones, and women after the menopause and the elderly require calcium to guard against osteoporosis, or brittle bones. Dairy products are one of the main sources of calcium, so if you fall into these categories and cut down on dairy products it may be advisable to take a calcium supplement every day.

Fresh fruit is a rich source of essential vitamins for all ages.

Allergy Diary

DATE	TIME EATEN OR DRUNK	FOOD/DRINK	ANY REACTION	TIME OF REACTION
10/9	7.30am	Toothpaste		
	7.45am	Bran flakes with milk and sugar Wholemeal toast with chocolate spread Orange juice		
		Coffee with milk and sugar		
			Slight itchiness of lips, 15 mins	9am
	11am	Tea with milk and sugar Digestive biscuits		
	12.30pm	Wholemeal bread cheese and salad sandwich, apple , mineral water		
	4pm	Tea with milk and sugar Chocolate bar		
			Mild stomach ache, 30 mins	6pm
	7pm	Cheese omelette with mixed salad White wine, Yoghurt		
	11pm	Milk drink		
		Toothpaste		

ELIMINATION DIETS

If you suspect that you are suffering from a food allergy (see pp. 30–33), it is vital that you identify the allergen responsible so that you can take steps to remove it from your diet – but only after consulting your doctor. An elimination diet will help identify the allergen, and then you can take steps to ensure that you do not expose yourself to it again (see pp. 106–107).

The first part of the process is mundane but essential: buy yourself a notebook. The aim is to use it to build up a body of information that may bring a pattern to light, and then to narrow the possibilities down until any allergen is positively identified. The information you record will also be valuable for any doctor or allergist whom you consult later.

At the front of the notebook, list any food and drink, record any physical symptom or change of mood, together with the time at which it occurs, how long it continues and the time at which it occurs (see above).

Leave a space at the bottom of each page to record more details of any symptoms, as well as a note of your bowel movements. How frequent are they? Are the stools well-formed or watery? Is there any unusual smell or colour?

Naturopathy

Naturopathy is ancient therapy – it goes back at least as far as the days of Hippocrates, the physician of ancient Greece – and the 'homeostasis', or equilibrium, that it stresses is similar in concept to that of the 'prana' of Ayurvedic medicine and the 'chi' of Chinese medicine. Naturopaths believe that nature is the healer of disease and that symptoms are an expression of the body's fight against any imbalance within it in an attempt to recover equilibrium. The imbalance that is causing the problem is the result of what naturopaths consider to be an 'unnatural' lifestyle: toxins build up in the body as a result of a bad diet, inadequate exercise and stress.

You can put the basic principles of preventive naturopathy into practice at home – the rules are those of common sense. To prevent a build-up of toxins, to remain healthy and to help prevent any allergic response from occurring you should make sure that you breathe fresh air, drink clean water, eat wholesome food, and take adequate exercise and rest.

SYMPTOMS ARE A HEALTHY SIGN

However, naturopaths believe that once a condition has developed, more active measures are needed. These are aimed not at relieving symptoms – which, after all, are only the outward signs of the body's attempt to rid itself of toxins – but at encouraging the body's own healing systems to flush out the toxins. In fact, the symptoms are considered a healthy sign, because they show that the body is fighting the toxins, and should be helped and encouraged to do so – in the same way that getting up a sweat helps cure a fever. Any aggressive treatment would put the body under more stress and make things worse, naturopaths believe, so they emphasize that any treatment should be gentle and take into account the whole person, considering his or her mental state and environment.

CONSULTING A NATUROPATH

In some countries, such as Germany, naturopaths have a similar standing to doctors and recommend that a number of treatments are tried alongside their own, such as hydrotherapy, herbalism, acupuncture, massage, chiropractic and homeopathy. Recognition of naturopathy lags behind in some other Western countries, but most now have recognized three- to four-year courses of study in the subject, which lead to a diploma or a degree. Contact the appropriate national organization to find the name of a qualified naturopath in your area *(see pp. 124–5)**.*

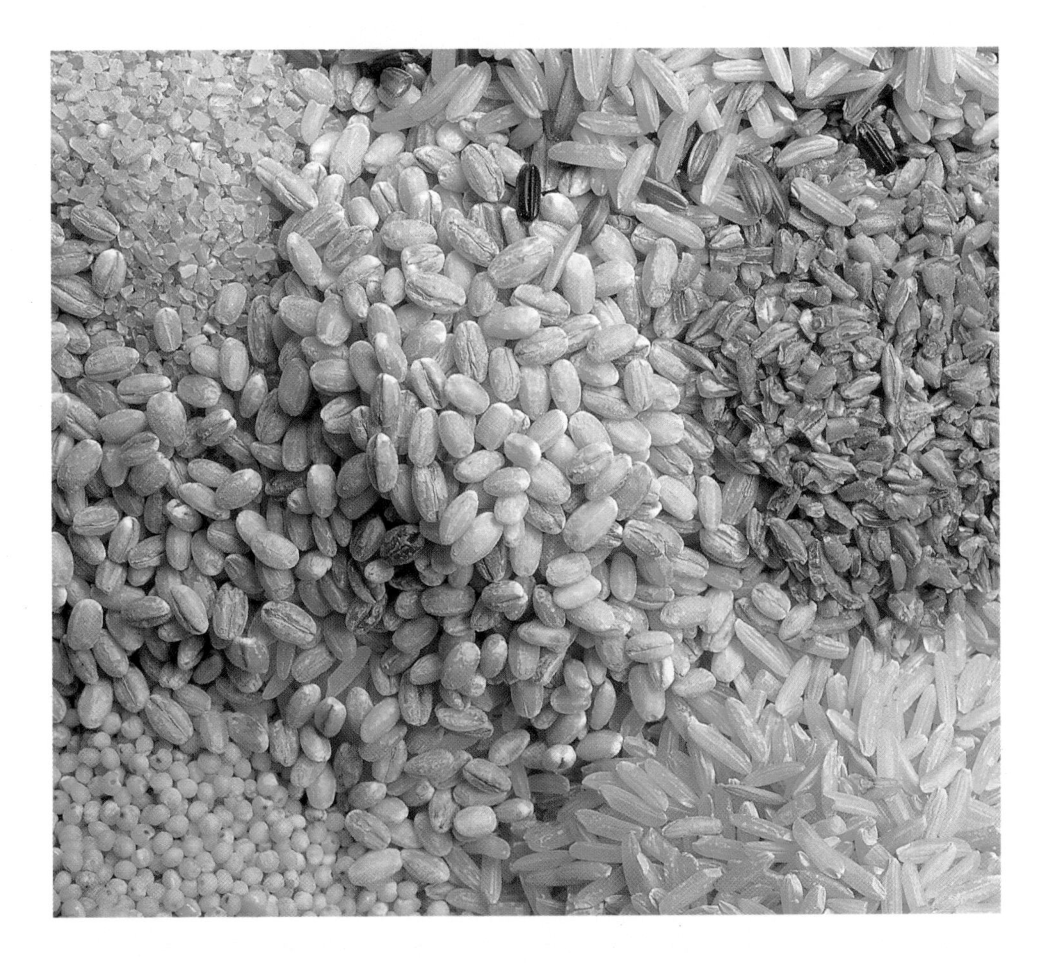

Unpolished rice and whole grains provide excellent natural fibre for a healthy diet.

FLUSHING OUT THE TOXINS

Naturopaths often advocate short fasts of two to three days, during which only vegetable and fruit juices are taken, to allow the body time to rest, in a physiological sense, and to boost the immune system in order to fight any toxins. They believe, too, that many modern ailments are the result of poor function of the bowels, and some naturopaths advocate the use of colonic irrigation. This practice can be dangerous, however, and the majority of naturopaths suggest colonic cleansing instead – the use of a high-fibre dietary supplement has a similar result and is safer and cheaper. After treatment, they stress the importance of a diet that is rich in unrefined foods and fibre.

MEDICAL WATCHPOINT

Do not attempt to fast for longer than two days unless you have consulted your doctor beforehand, and do not stop taking any medically prescribed drugs without consultation. This is especially important if you have any pre-existing medical condition.

Herbal remedies

The human race evolved in close communion with the world of plants. Plants have always been a staple part of our diet, and the healing effects of some – and toxic effects of others – must have become apparent to our earliest ancestors. It is hardly surprising that herbs and plant extracts have formed the basis of the healing arts for thousands of years. Every civilization has at some time developed a system of herbal medicine, and in some parts of the world, for example China, these traditional systems are still very much in use. Nobody would deny that modern medicine has saved untold numbers of lives and has enabled us to live longer and to enjoy better health, but modern medicine does not have all the answers. And, increasingly, people – including pharmaceutical companies – are realising that the herbal wisdom of our ancestors still has much to offer.

Herbal remedies can be useful in both preventing the onset of an allergic reaction and in relieving its symptoms. In the following pages you will find suggestions for preparing and using some common and simple herbal preparations – herbal teas, decoctions, tinctures and inhalations – known to be helpful for those suffering from asthma, hayfever and other allergies. However, to take full advantage of the power of herbal medicine, whether Western or Oriental, you should consult an experienced herbalist, who will consider all aspects of your life before deciding which preparations would be best for you and your condition.

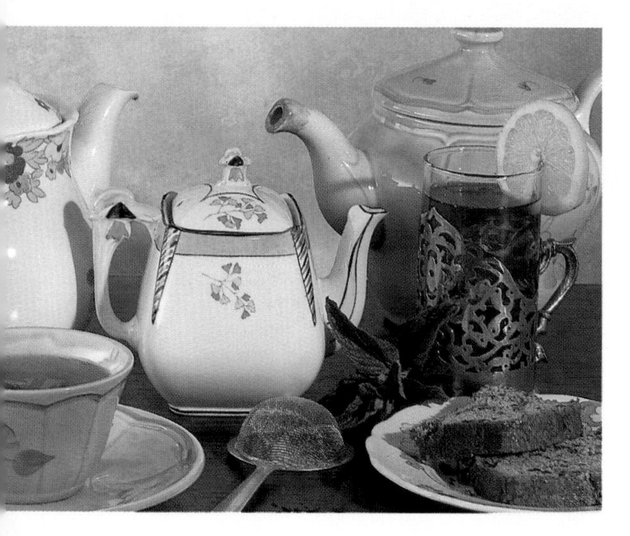

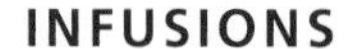

INFUSIONS

Infusion is the usual way of making a herbal tea – a delightfully refreshing way of taking a herbal remedy, and one that makes the herb easy to assimilate and digest.

Chop fresh or dried herbs finely, and blend in a pestle and mortar. Put them in a warm china teapot, and add boiling water. Cover and allow to rest for 1–3 minutes in the case of flowers, and for

Herbal teas or infusions can easily be incorporated into a daily routine.

2–4 minutes if you are using leaves. Strain into a teacup. Do not keep the infusion for more than a few hours. Milk tends to suppress the flavour of herb teas, but a spoon of honey or a few drops of lemon juice can enhance it.

Dosage: one cup, three to six times a day. Pause to inhale the aroma before drinking, because this in itself has healing properties.

DECOCTIONS

Use a decoction to make a herbal tea if the plant material you have consists of hard parts, such as bark or seeds.

Chop and crush the ingredients as finely as you can. Place them in a saucepan – non-stick is best – and cover with water. Cover and bring slowly to the boil. Allow to simmer for 10–15 minutes, then strain into a teapot. Use as for an infusion, throwing unused decoction away after a few hours

Dosage: as for infusions.

TINCTURES

Unlike infusions and decoctions, tinctures can be stored more or less indefinitely. Tinctures are highly concentrated herbal extracts mixed with alcohol. If you don't want to drink alcohol, you can pour the dose into a quarter of a cup of water before you take it and leave it uncovered for a few hours to allow the alcohol to evaporate.

Chop or bruise the herb. To make 200–300ml (7–10fl oz) of tincture you will need 15g (1/2oz) of dried herbs or 30g (1oz) of fresh herbs. Put the herb into a large jar and add a mixture of 200ml (7fl oz) of alcohol, such as vodka or brandy, and 85ml (3fl oz) of water. Seal the jar, label it and leave to stand in a cool, dark place for two weeks, turning it upside-down daily. Strain through a loose-weave cotton cloth placed in a strainer, and discard the spent herbs. Pour the strained liquid into clean, dark coloured glass bottles and label them.

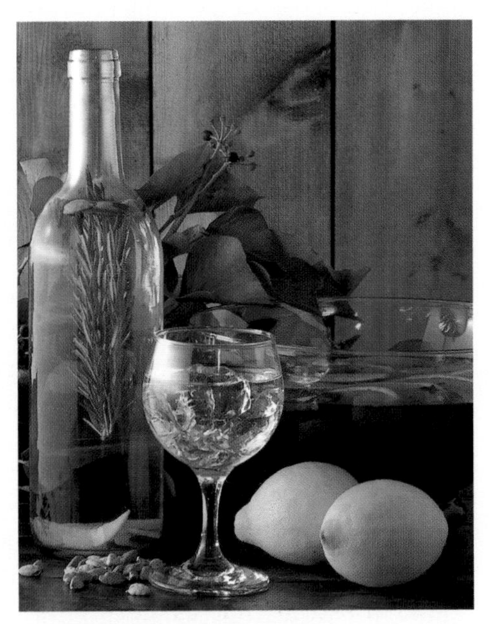

Tinctures are herbal extracts concentrated in alcohol, a good method for long-term keeping – but always remember to label the bottle.

SYRUPS

Syrups are the basis of many cough remedies, and generally help thin out mucus and open up the airways.

Chop 40g (1 1/2oz) of herb and place in a pan with 900ml (1 1/2pt) of water. Bring to the boil, cover and simmer on a low heat for 20 minutes. Allow the liquid to cool and strain into another pan, squeezing the herbs with a spoon to extract all the goodness. Then return the strained liquid to the heat and simmer gently until it has reduced to 200ml (7fl oz). Add 450g (1lb) of sugar or honey to the pan, and simmer for a few minutes, stirring all the time until the liquid has the consistency of syrup – don't let the mixture overheat. Take off the heat, allow the syrup to cool and store it in clean bottles.

Dosage (also for tinctures): for children, one teaspoon, 3–6 times daily; for adults, two teaspoons, 3-6 times daily

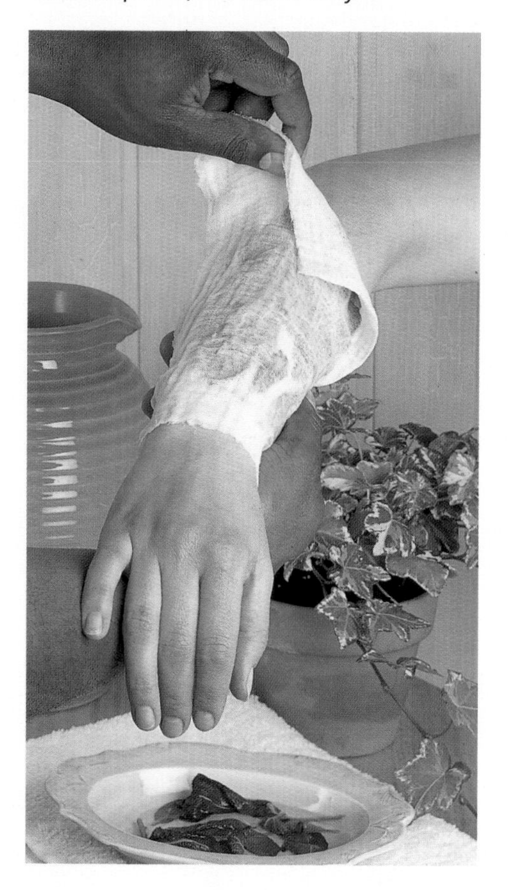

COMPRESSES AND POULTICES

Compresses and poultices provide a way of applying herbal infusions and decoctions directly to the skin – to reduce inflammation or itching, for example, or to prevent infection in a wound or raw patch of skin.

Make an infusion or decoction according to the instructions already given. Soak a soft, clean cloth in the warm liquid and apply it to the affected area. This is a compress. Alternatively, make a poultice by taking the mushy residue of herbal material from an infusion and wrap it in a piece of gauze. Apply this to the affected area and cover with a dry cloth to retain the warmth.

INHALATIONS

Respiratory complaints, including asthma and hayfever, can benefit from inhalation. The steam has a soothing effect on the airways and nasal passages, and the steam can be used to deliver a dose of herbal medicine.

Herbal infusions and decoctions made in a bowl can be used for inhaling. Alternatively, a few drops of tincture, or aromatherapy oils, can be added to just-boiled water. Bend over the bowl and cover your head, shoulders and the bowl with a towel. Breathe in the steam through your nose for about 20 minutes. Reheat in a saucepan halfway through the process to keep up a good supply of steam.

A herbal poultice can be an effective method for soothing the inflammation of an allergic skin condition.

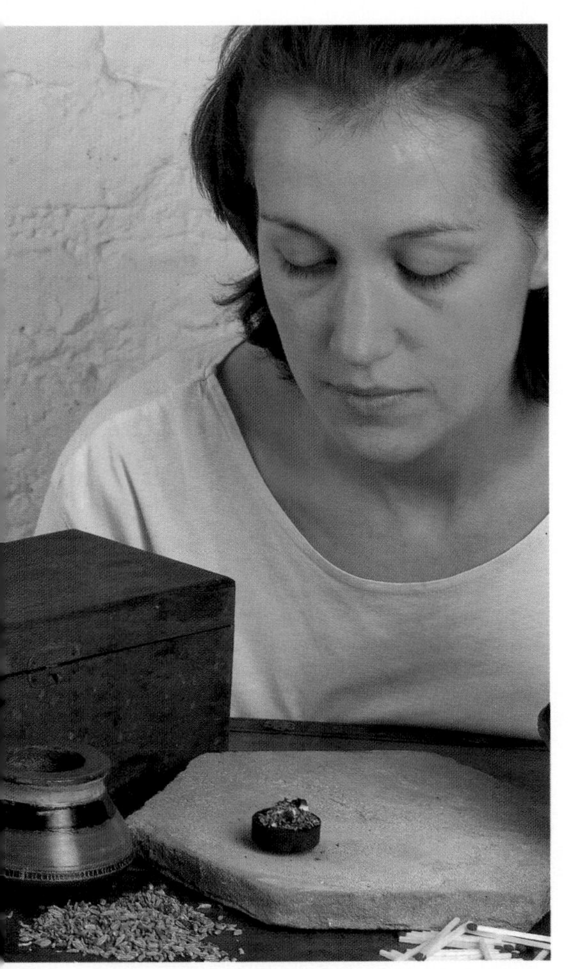

Pastilles of compressed herbs can be made as inhalants. When lit, the pastilles smoulder, and the smoke is inhaled.

THE HERBS TO USE

Because allergic symptoms are so diverse, herbal treatments concentrate on particular allergies rather than on treating hypersensitivity as a whole – although there is good evidence that the Chinese herb Ma Huang (*Ephedra*) can be used for a wide range of allergic conditions. Here are a few of the tried and tested remedies for the different allergic conditions.

ASTHMA

***Althaea officinalis* (marsh mallow root)** – soothes and relaxes the air passages and stimulates the immune system; take as a decoction or tincture.

***Eucalyptus* (eucalyptus oil)** – an antiseptic and decongestant; take as an inhalation.

***Glycyrrhiza glabra* (liquorice root)** – an anti-inflammatory that stimulates the adrenal glands; chew a piece or take as a decoction.

***Inula helenium* (elecampane)** – take as an infusion or inhalation (see Hayfever below).

***Matricaria recutita* (chamomile)** – an anti-inflammatory containing natural antihistamine; take as an infusion or inhalation.

***Tussilago farfara* (coltsfoot)** – an anticatarrhal and expectorant; take as an infusion of flowers and leaves.

***Verbascum thapsus* (mullein)** – an anti-inflammatory and soothing to the air passages; take as an infusion or apply infused oils to the skin for eczema.

ECZEMA

***Arctium lappa* (burdock)** – an anti-inflammatory and antibiotic; use as a decoction of roots, particularly for weeping eczema, or apply a poultice of the leaves directly to the skin.

***Calendula officinalis* (marigold)** – an anti-inflammatory that strengthens the immune system: take as an infusion, or apply infused oil directly to the skin.

Hypericum perforatum **(St John's wort)** – an anti-inflammatory often used for skin conditions; apply the infused oil directly to the skin.

Stellaria media **(chickweed)** – See Hives

HAYFEVER

Allium sativum **(garlic)** – an antibiotic and antihistamine; use in cooking or in capsule form.

Euphrasia officinalis **(eyebright)** – a decongestant that soothes the mucous membranes and conjunctiva; take as an infusion or tincture, or use diluted to rinse the eyes.

Inula helenium **(elecampane)** – a stimulant that relieves respiratory ailments; take regularly as a decoction of the roots, or use to bathe the skin for eczema.

Urticaria urens **(nettle)** – an anti-inflammatory and anti-allergic; eat the leaves boiled as a vegetable or in soups, or drink as an infusion.

HIVES (URTICARIA)

Matricaria recutite **(chamomile)** – use as a compress or poultice to relieve itching (see Asthma above).

Stellaria media (chickweed) – an astringent and anti-irritant; take as an infusion, or apply directly to the skin as a cream.

CHINESE HERBAL MEDICINE

The popularity of Chinese herbal medicine has been growing in the last few years. In China itself it is widely respected and officially recognized as the heir to a tradition that goes back nearly 5000 years. Although both Western and Chinese herbal medicine share a belief in the potency of herbal remedies, they differ in basic philosophy and in practice.

At the heart of Chinese herbal medicine lies the belief that illness results from imbalance or disharmony in the elements that control the body. Where ancient Western medicine held there to be four basic elements (earth, air, fire and water), the Chinese count five (wood, fire, earth, metal and water). Each of these elements exists in a distinct relationship with another; problems in parts of the body represented by wood (the liver, for example) might be due to deficiencies in the parts represented by water (the kidneys). In addition, Chinese herbal medicine incorporates the concepts of yin and yang, where yin represents the female principle and is seen as dark and cold, while yang represents the male principle and is seen as light and hot. All these elements must be in balance if good health is to be maintained.

As a result, Chinese herbal medicine is extremely subtle. Where Western herbal medicine uses individual herbs or a limited number of herbs in combination, Chinese remedies often contain many ingredients, mixed in very precise proportions. Remedies for sufferers from allergic conditions are plentiful, but

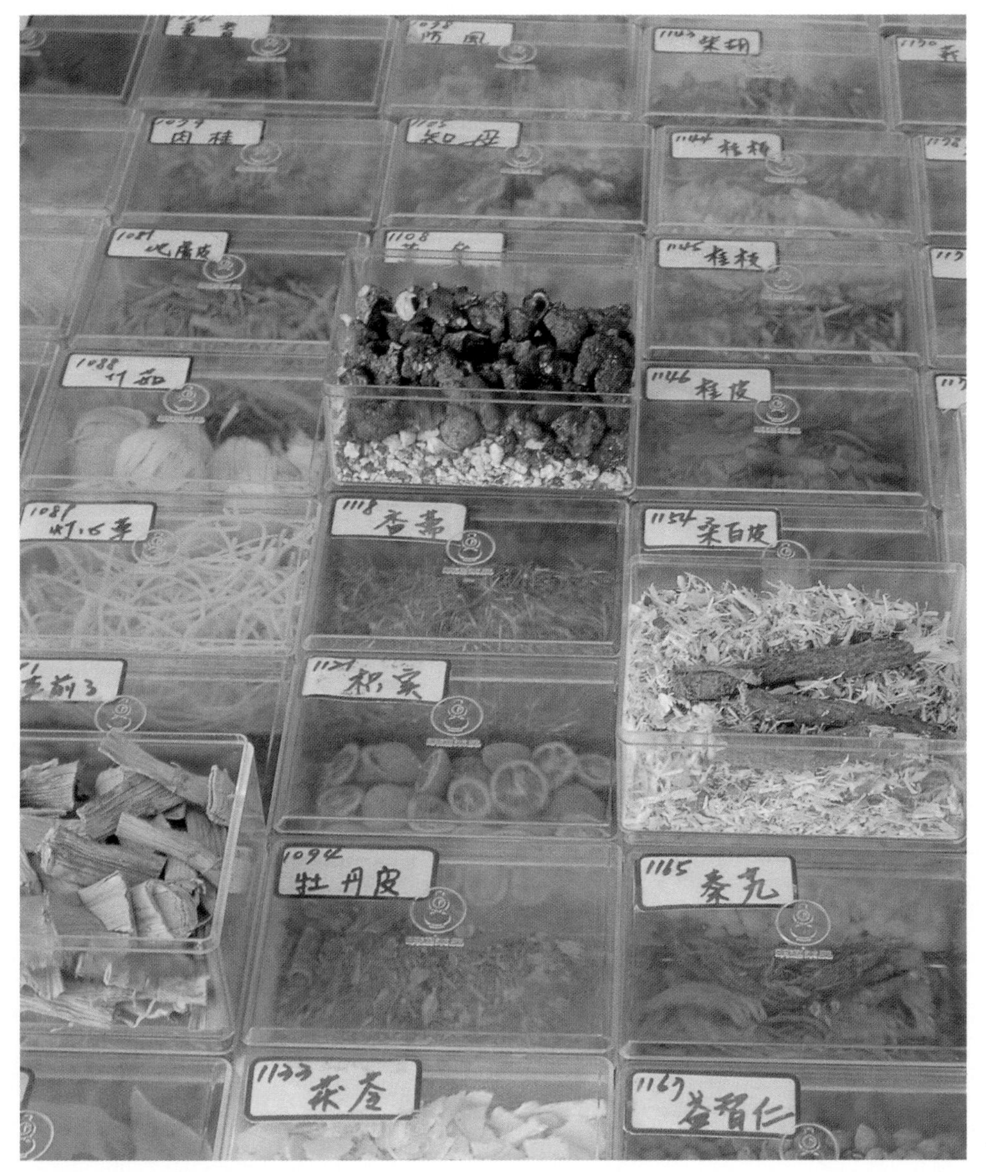

Chinese medicinal herbs seen in a medical factory in Taiwan. In Chinese culture, herbal practitioners are highly respected as the heirs to thousands of years of tradition.

most of them contain Ma Huang (known in the West as *Ephedra*), combined with such other herbs as astragalus, liquorice and ginger. The use of *Ephedra* is restricted in some countries, including the UK, Australia and New Zealand, because of its potency, and can only be acquired from a registered practitioner. However, you should consult a qualified practitioner in any case if you want to test the benefits of this ancient and sophisticated system of healing.

Homeopathy

Some 200 years ago, Samuel Hahnemann, a German physician and chemist, analysed the results of his observations and of experiments on himself and came up with 'The Law of Similars – that is, a remedy can cure a disease if it produces symptoms similar to those of the disease in a healthy person. His work was the groundstone of what was to become homeopathy.

The trouble was that the use of such remedies caused inevitable side-effects since they triggered symptoms. But after further experiment, Hahnemann found that a considerable dilution of the remedy not only eliminated side-effects, but made the remedy more effective. He claimed this effect as the principle of the 'Minimum Dose', and called the way in which it worked 'potentization'.

Today, homeopathic medicine is well-established worldwide, and its efficacy is accepted by many practitioners of conventional medicine. It is not simply used as a treatment for specific conditions but also as a general strengthening agent for the immune system, so homeopathic treatments can be used as a preventive measure against allergies in general and against hayfever in particular. However, choosing the correct treatment for this purpose involves consideration of a number of factors and is best undertaken on a long-term basis by a qualified homeopath. However, they should not be used as a substitute for medical treatment in the case of an acute allergic response: their function is primarily preventive.

Nevertheless, there are several specific homeopathic treatments for hayfever and for insect bites to which there is only a minor response. They can be bought at most health stores, though you will also need to buy a few bottles of lactose (milk sugar) carrier pills, some pure alcohol, a test-tube stand and test tubes and a pipette. The next step is to make up the remedies, by dilution and re-dilution – which as well as increasing their effect, ensures that they can be given to anyone, of any age, without danger.

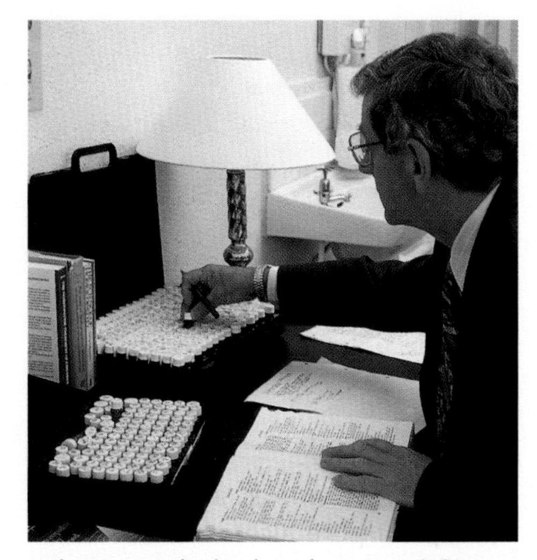

A homeopath checks tubes containing homeopathic medicine.

MAKING A HOMEOPATHIC REMEDY

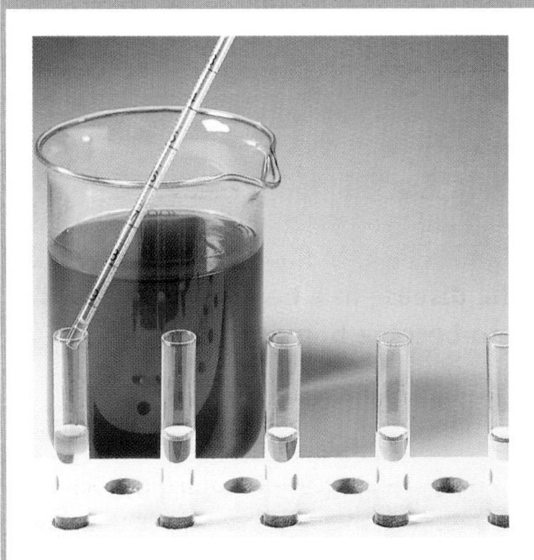

MAKING THE REMEDIES

The first step is to produce a 'tincture', by soaking the plant material in pure alcohol for a few weeks. Once this 'mother tincture' is ready, it is time to start diluting the tincture to the correct potency. In the case of these hayfever remedies, this should be '6x' – meaning that it has been diluted six times, each dilution being in a ratio of one drop of the previous liquid to nine drops of pure alcohol. Between after each dilution, the mixture is shaken vigorously by knocking it against the palm of the hand, in a process known as 'succussation'.

MAKING A 6X POTENCY

1 Making sure that the remedy is of the correct potency is not a difficult procedure, but accuracy is required. First of all, set six test tubes up in a rack, and place nine drops of pure alcohol in each. You will need a pipette and a bottle of lactose (milk sugar) carrier pills at hand.

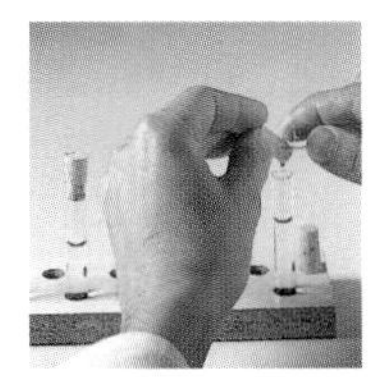

2 Measure one drop – of the same size used for the drops of alcohol – of the mother tincture and place it in the first test-tube: you now have a 1x potency remedy.

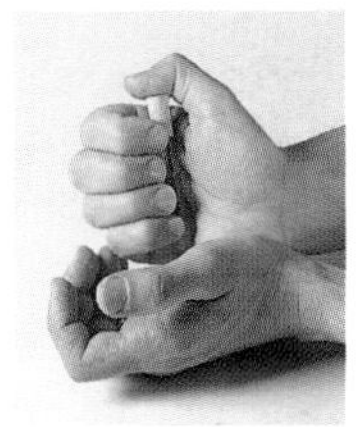

3 Succuss the liquid to mix it thoroughly by knocking the test-tube against the palm of your hand.

4 Place one drop of the 1x mixture from the first tube into the second tube, and succuss again. Repeat the process with the next four tubes.

5 Now at 6x potency, the mixture can be added to the bottle of lactose carrier pills, and the homeopathic remedy is complete.

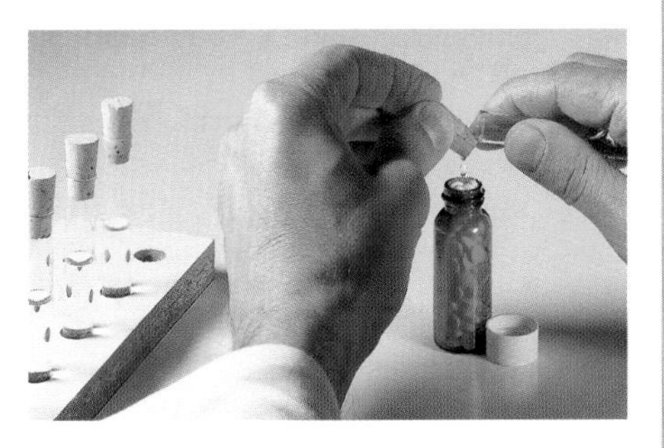

Taking the remedies

Homeopathy practice stresses that only one remedy should be taken at a time, so choose the one that is the most appropriate for the symptoms that are predominant in you and try that first.

Allium cepa (red onion)

Try this remedy, at 6x potency, when:

- you sneeze frequently;
- you have a heavy, burning discharge from the nose;
- your eyes secrete a bland, watery fluid;
- the smell of flowers aggravates the symptoms.

Dosage (all remedies): one dose every two to four hours for two days, then reduce to three times daily for a further three to five days.

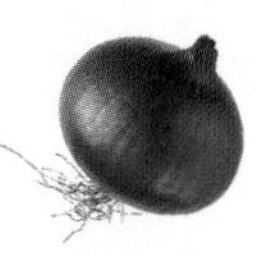

Allium cepa (red onion)

Ambrosia

Try this remedy, at 6x potency, when:

- your nose is dripping and your eyes are itching after exposure to ragweed (ambrosia is a homeopathic dose of ragweed).

Apis mellifica (honeybee venom)

Try this remedy, at 6x potency, when:

- your throat is swollen and puffy;
- your skin feels tight and sensitive to the touch (you may have hives as well);
- or when you have a red, inflamed insect bite and its irritation is relieved by cold.

STORING HOMEOPATHIC REMEDIES

Remedies will keep well if you observe some basic precautions:

- *keep them in the dark, away from heat sources, and try to touch them as little as possible as they can be spoiled by heat and light;*
- *keep them away from any strong-smelling products, such as perfume, mothballs and aromatherapy oils;*
- *never put remedies in old containers, because traces of any original remedy will adhere to them.*

***Arsenicum* (white oxide of metallic arsenic)**

Try this remedy, at 6x potency, when:

- you have burning tears and a discharge from your nose that is worse on the right side of your face;
- you are restless at night;
- you are very thirsty;
- you are sensitive to light and your chest is tight.

***Euphrasia* (eyebright)**

Try this remedy, at 6x potency, when:

- your eyes are red, burning, watery and itchy;
- any nasal discharge is bland;
- your symptoms become worse in sunlight and the warmth and worse in open air.

NB Euphrasia can also be taken externally, in the form of eyedrops. Use drops of the mother tincture for this purpose.

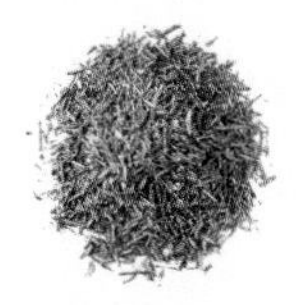

Euphrasia (eyebright)

***Ledum* (wild rosemary)**

Try this remedy, at 6x potency, when:

- have a mosquito bite or insect sting that is itching and the irritation is relieved by cold.

***Nux vomica* (posion nut)**

Try this remedy, at 6x potency, when:

- you have a dripping nose during the day and are congested at night;
- your symptoms are better out of doors, and worse indoors.

***Pulsillata* (meadow anemone, pasque flower, wind flower)**

Try this remedy, at 6x potency, when:

- your nose runs during the day but is congested during the night, which becomes worse in the warm;
- feel moody;
- the roof of your mouth itches at night.

Sabadilla

Try this remedy, at 6x potency, when:

- you have an itchy nose, red eyes and a headache;
- you feel that you have a lump in your throat.

Flower remedies

The idea that flowers have the power to alter emotional states has been around for a long time – the indigenous populations of America and Australia used flowers as part of their armoury of herbal remedies. But it was not until the 1920s that Dr Edward Bach (pronounced 'Batch'), a pathologist and bacteriologist working in London's Harley Street, devised the system that takes his name. His Flower Remedies are not treatments for an acute allergic response, but they have their place in fortifying body and spirit, so that the body – through the mind – is best prepared to ward off the effects of such a response. Today, the interest in complementary flower remedies continues to grow.

Bach believed that many of his patients suffered from negative emotional states and that these either caused or aggravated the physical symptoms of which they complained. Becoming disenchanted with the conventional medicine of the day, which tended to treat symptoms rather than the cause of a disease, he retired to a cottage in Wales to search for a new system of healing that would alter negative emotional states.

Bach found that the dew found on certain flowers affected his own feelings, and he experimented further by creating a negative emotional state within his own mind and then testing the dew from various flowers to see which ones had a positive effect. The outcome was his system of flower remedies, consisting of remedies for 38 distinct emotional states.

Bach believed that his remedies work in two ways: they stimulate the body's own healing powers; and they encourage one to combat a negative emotional state in a positive way. As far as allergies are concerned, they can help keep the psyche calm and well-balanced, creating the ideal conditions for the immune system to work to its full potential.

A selection of Bach Flower Remedies, intended to promote healing through positive mood control.

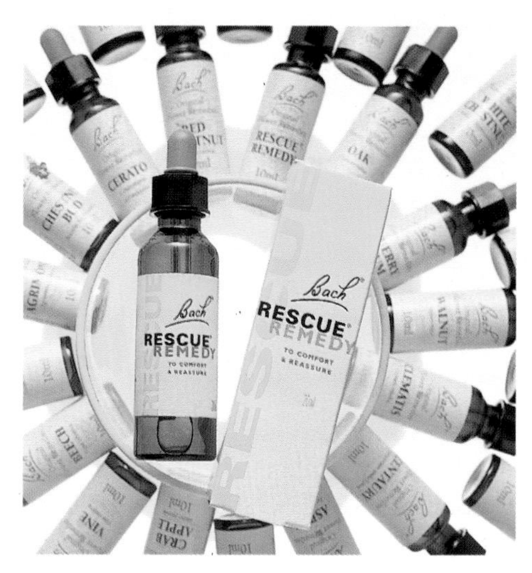

NEW FLOWER REMEDIES

Clare Harvey, a published expert on flower remedies and vibrational medicine, has noted a 'veritable explosion' of modern interest in healing with flower essences in the wake of Bach's pioneering work. Since the essences have no chemical constituents, Clare Harvey believes that they must work positively with the body's natural healing system. She lists a selection of flower essence remedies for allergy-sensitive people. Names in brackets are those of the manufacturers:

Asthma

Babies' Breath (Petite Fleur) Eases congestion in the lungs, aids asthma, *Eucalyptus* (FES) clears congestion and soothes inflammation in the lungs, sinuses and nasal passages.
Grape Hyacinth (Pacific) For times of external shock and stress; dissolves shock, aiding breathing.

Food allergies

Green Rose (FES) For the condition that can lead to allergic responses to certain food, also for migraines and hayfever.

Hayfever

Green Rose (FES) as above
Lantana (Petite Fleur) For the quiet, over-sensitive types who are prone to allergens, hayfever sufferers.
Bush Iris and *Dagger Hakea* (Aus Bush) combined for relief of hayfever.

Insect stings

Garlic (FES) Excellent for poor immune response and vulnerability to infection, offers relief to insect stings.

Skin allergies

Luffa (FES) Cleanser, if an internal problem is creating a skin condition; treats most skin conditions, eg eczema.
Lily plus Salvia (Petite Fleur) For anxiety and fear, especially about the future and not being in control. This boosts the immune system and aids skin allergies.
Vanilla Leaf (Pacific) Works on the lungs and colon, for skin disorders that are rooted in low self-esteem.

Immune boosters

Gaillarda (Petite Fleur) Galvanizes the immune system to dissolve invaders. Boosts immunity by enhancing resistance.
Snapdragon (Petite Fleur) Enhances the internal and external judgement and discernment, raising the consciousness of the immune system

Anti-stress remedies

Macrocarpa (Aus Bush) For exhaustion resulting in poor immune resistance.
White Carnation (Petite Fleur) For tension and anxiety.

Sensitivity to the environment

Pink Fairy Orchid (Aus Living) For those who can become panicky due to feeling overwhelmed by circumstance. Filters out the stress and helps to lessen over-sensitivity to the environment.

Natural rescuersF

Pear Blossom (Masters) Ideal for any situation which throws one off balance; helps stabilize emergencies.
Five Flower Remedy (Healing Herbs) A rescue essence that boosts the whole system.

Acupuncture

Acupuncture was developed in China as long as 5000 years ago, but its introduction into the West is relatively recent. Initial interest in the technique in the early nineteenth century faded, as more and more advances were made in conventional medicine. Then, in 1973, the Royal Society for Medicine in Britain published a survey showing that 37 per cent of a sample of people suffering from apparently intractable diseases were 'cured or much improved' after acupuncture. In particular, though, four out of five hayfever sufferers found that their condition had improved. It was this survey that led to what is now a widespread acceptance of acupuncture as a viable alternative treatment for many conditions, including allergies.

The cornerstone of acupuncture is the belief that disease is the result of imbalance between the female and the male principles – 'yin' and 'yang' – in the body. This affects the flow of the body's vital energy – 'chi' or 'qi' – along a series of pathways called meridians. An expert acupuncturist hopes to restore the body's essential harmony by manipulating the flow of energy at the sites, called acupoints, where these meridians are closest to the skin.

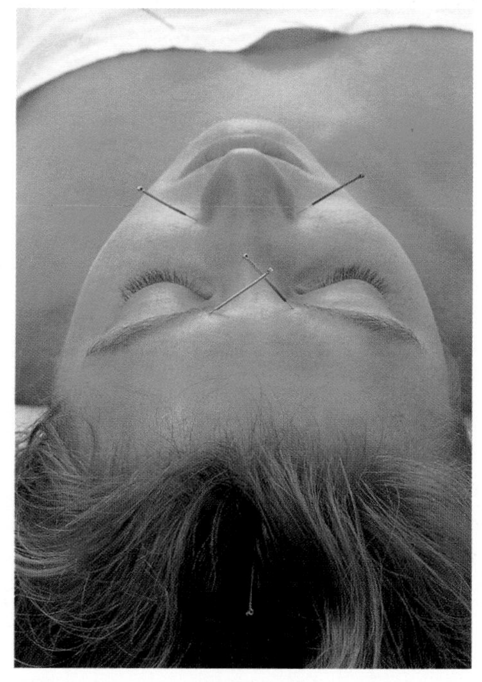

This patient is undergoing acupuncture treatment for hayfever. Needles are inserted into the skin of the face at points on the bladder and large intestine meridians. The acupuncturist hopes to correct 'imbalances' in the body which cause the symptoms.

Western medicine rejects the basic philosophy of Chinese acupuncture but accepts that it can work. There are a number of theories as to why this might be. One is that acupuncture blocks the transmission of pain signals at the spinal cord – but this does not explain how it is effective in the treatment of conditions such as hayfever and arthritis. Another is that acupuncture stimulates the production of endorphins, the body's natural painkillers. There are also some surprising coincidences between the practice of acupuncture and Western medicine. Many acupoints are located where nerves emerge from the deep tissues towards the skin; also, 71 per cent of acupoints correspond to 'trigger points' – areas on the skin that become tender in certain diseases, such as the pain that is felt in the shoulder from liver disease.

Most people tend to visit an acupuncturist only when conventional medical treatments have failed. However, given that the technique has a proven track record with allergies, you may well decide to visit a registered acupuncturist at an early stage (see pp. 124–5). Be warned, however: as acupuncturists themselves admit, acupuncture is ineffective on around one in four people.

VISITING AN ACUPUNCTURIST

An essential preliminary in any consultation with an acupuncturist is taking your pulse. This provides vital information about any imbalances that may be present in your body. The Nei Ching, the first textbook of acupuncture, compiled between 479 and 300BC, describes the 12 pulses that must be examined – six in each wrist. Western practitioners may offer a simplified form of the traditional procedure.

Once the diagnosis has been made, the acupuncturist will insert silver alloy or stainless steel needles with great precision into any of the 365 acupoints in the body (600 according to one school of acupuncture) in order to adjust the balance of energy that flows along the meridians. The needles are round-tipped, with the result that they divide the flesh rather than pierce it, so there is rarely any blood. Then the needles are delicately twirled or pumped gently up and down by the acupuncturist to stimulate the flow of chi.

Acupuncture directed solely at the ear is known as auricular therapy. It is based on the notion that the ear is a mirror of the body as a whole and that manipulation of the more than 120 acupoints on each ear can therefore treat almost any disorder.

Moxibustion is another ancient technique related to acupuncture, in which sticks of the herb *Moxa* (mugwort) are burned close to the meridian points on the skin, or alternatively, they may be burned onto the needles used for conventional acupuncture.

In the West, a number of techniques have been introduced to enhance the traditional method of manual manipulation. Most of these involve the use of electricity, either as a means of determining the flow of energy through the meridians and so deciding the exact acupoints that need treatment, or as way of delivering small electric currents to the acupuncture needles themselves to help improve circulation. Some acupuncturists have also experimented with the use of lasers to stimulate the acupoints directly. Others have tried combining acupuncture with herbal extracts or sound.

Acupressure

Acupressure is acupuncture without needles. It is based on the same principles as acupuncture (see pp. 72–73) and has the same aim of restoring the flow of healing energy – chi – along special pathways in the body, called meridians, but it uses finger pressure and gentle massage to achieve its effects. Acupressure is also an essential element in the ancient Japanese technique called shiatsu. It is an ideal self-help treatment, although you will need a partner to work on some of the pressure points.

Acupressure has been shown to be effective in the treatment of most types of allergy. Combined with breathing exercises (see pp. 20–21) and other forms of relaxation, it can reduce the severity of an attack of asthma; it can help clear the congestion and painful sinuses associated with hayfever; it can reduce the itchiness of urticaria; and it may have long-term benefits in reducing sensitivity in eczema.

Acupressure points are usually quite easy to find, since they are often marked by a slight indentation in the skin and may feel slightly more sensitive than the surrounding area. The illustrations on pp. 76–7 show which ones are suitable for the treatment of allergic symptoms. However, these are not the only points that may be effective, because everyone has their personal 'tender spots', known as 'ah shi'. These are often found around the head, neck and face. so it is worth experimenting to find your own.

ACUPRESSURE IN PRACTICE

The rule with acupressure is 'a little and often' – around five times a day, every day, for several minutes at a time if you can manage it.

Use the the ball of your thumb and the first and second fingers – take care not to dig into the skin with your fingernails.

Keep the pressure steady and even, increasing it gradually to a weight of about 450g (1lb) – use some kitchen scales to get an idea of this. Hold for about 20 seconds, then release slowly and gently; wait for about 10 seconds, then repeat for up to five times.

If your thumbs become tired, place your first finger on top of your middle finger – flattening it so that the nails do not touch the skin – and press with this instead.

Once you have mastered the technique, try making small circular movements, working clockwise, as you apply the pressure.

ACUPRESSURE, SHIATSU AND DO IN

Acupressure should not be confused with shiatsu. Shiatsu is a Japanese

Acupressure, like acupuncture, has long-established roots in traditional Chinese medicine. Pressure is applied by the hand or fingers to certain points in order to treat physical illness in another part of the body.

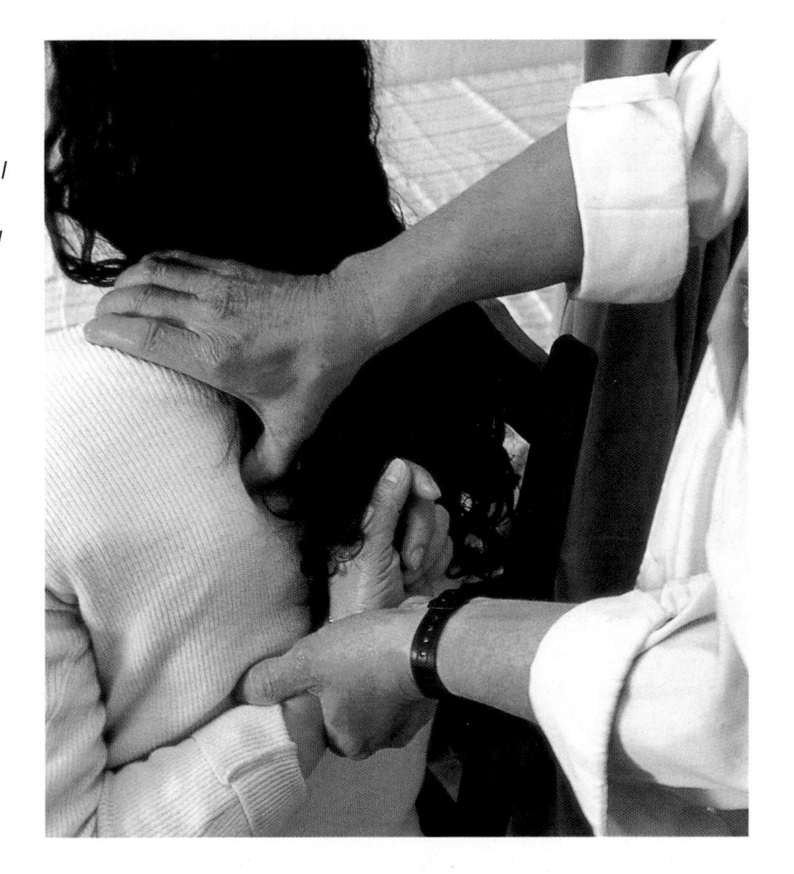

technique that developed separately after ancient Chinese massage techniques had been exported to Japan. Although the term does actually mean 'finger pressure', Shiatsu involves the use of knuckles, elbows, knees and feet in addition to fingers. It also mixes acu-pressure with a form of physio-therapy, along with osteopathy and exercise regimes. It should be undertaken by a specialist practitioner: it is not a self-help technique.

A self-help form of acupressure that has recently increased in popularity is the ancient Japanese system of Do In. This combines acupressure – concentrating on the face – with simple breathing and stretching exercises and with relaxation and meditation techniques. Many people find Do In a good way to start the day.

Other forms of acupressure concentrate entirely on the hands or, more often, the feet. Foot reflexology, in particular, is a very well established and sophisticated technique (see pp. 78–81).

MEDICAL WATCHPOINT

Make sure that you keep the amount of pressure used under careful control. You should never feel any pain – if you do, the treatment is being counter-productive.

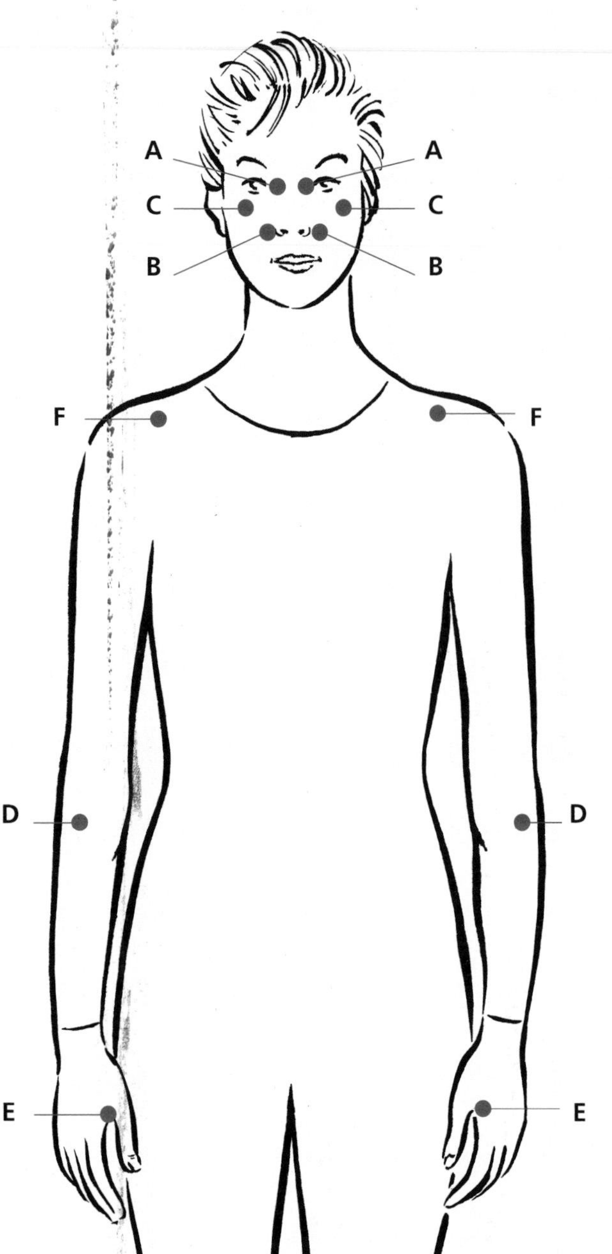

For hayfever, sinus and cold symptoms

Point A This is located just in front of the tear duct, on either side of the nose: also effective for tired eyes.

Point B This is located where the base of the nostril joins the face in the small groove on either side of the nose: also effective for toothache

Point C This is located on the point of the cheekbone, on either side of the face.

Point D This is located on the muscle of the inner forearm, three finger widths below the crease of the elbow and slightly to the outside of the centre line: good for general well-being.

Point E This is located in the webbing between the finger and the thumb on the front of the hand, at the point where the thumb joins the finger: also good for headache, toothache and other pain.

For asthma and other lung and chest complaints.

Point F This is located in the grooves between the upper ribs on either side of the breastbone.

MEDICAL WATCHPOINT

Make sure that you keep the amount of pressure used under careful control. You should never feel any pain – if you do, the treatment is being counterproductive.

Take particular care when applying pressure to pressure points at the base of the skull.

Always consult an acupressurist before beginning treatment if you are pregnant, taking medication, or suffering from a medical condition.

For sinus and cold symptoms

Point A This is located in the midline, in the indentation at the base of the skull at the top of the neck. Press up gently, as if into the skull: also good for headaches, stiff necks and nosebleeds.

Point B This is located just to the right and slightly higher than A on each side of the base of the skull. Feel for the indentation on each side of the mid-line, and push gently up and in: also good for headaches.

For asthma and other lung and chest complaints.

Point C This is located on the muscles that run down on either side of the spine, and between the shoulder blades: also good for strengthening the heart.

For stomach and digestive complaints.

Point D This is located below point C, on the muscles that run down on either side of the spine.

Point E This is located at the centre of the crease at the back of the knee; also good for relaxation and the relief of tension.

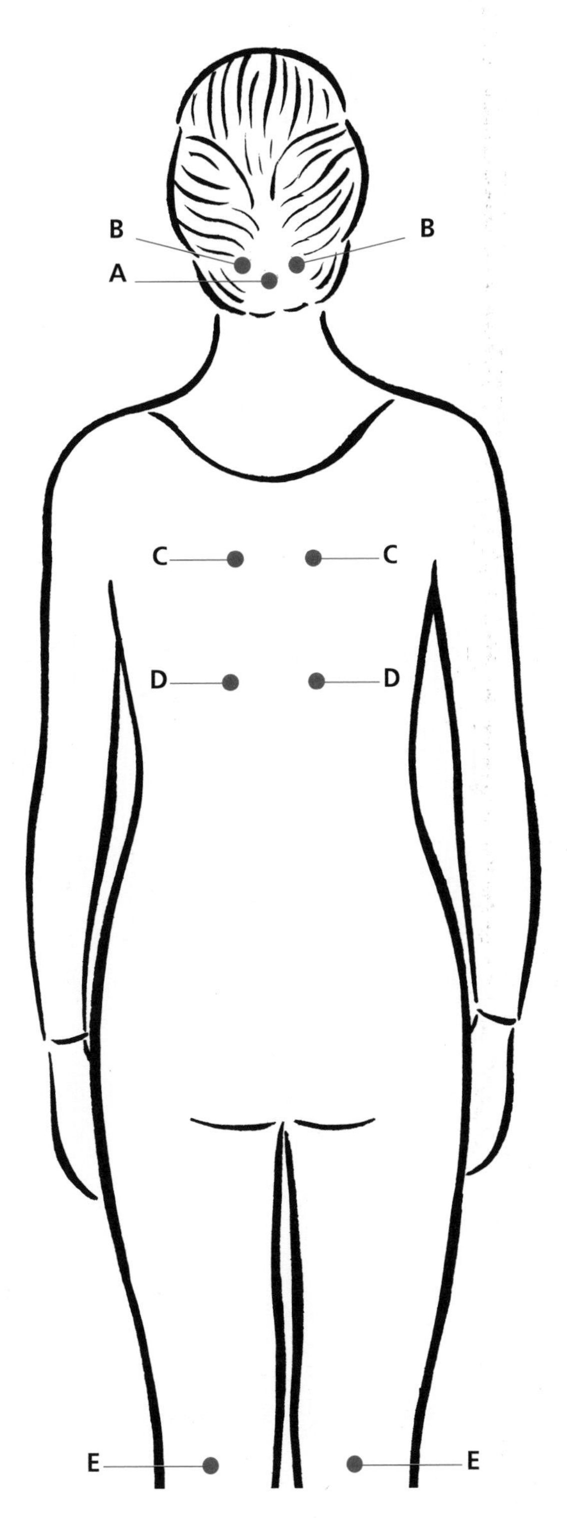

WARNING

It is dangerous to use too much pressure on the pressure points at the base of the skull: stop immediately if any light-headedness is experienced

Reflexology

Also called zone therapy and reflex zone therapy, reflexology is a healing system that works on the principle that the body's vital energy – chi – flows through 10 vertical channels down the body, and that the flow is blocked or disturbed as part of an illness. The channels end at the hands, ears and feet, but reflexologists concentrate on the feet because the points on which they work are nearer to the skin in the feet, which also provides a larger area on which to work. In addition, because the feet are termination points for the energy channels, they form a map of areas and organs of the body: each channel termination represents the parts of the body through which the channel passes.

By stimulating one of a number of precise points, reflexologists free the energy channel in which they are contained and so treat any tissue or organ through which the channel passes. At the same time, any point on the foot that is tender to the touch represents a problem elsewhere in the body, either latent or apparent, which means that reflexology is a preventive as well as remedial therapy.

There is no scientific proof of the theory of reflexology, but it does appear to be successful in the treatment of a number of conditions in practice – often in combination with other complementary techniques, such as osteopathy, acupressure, homeopathy and naturopathy. To gain the full benefit of reflexology, it is best to consult an experienced reflexologist. Unfortunately, however, no qualifications are needed to set up in

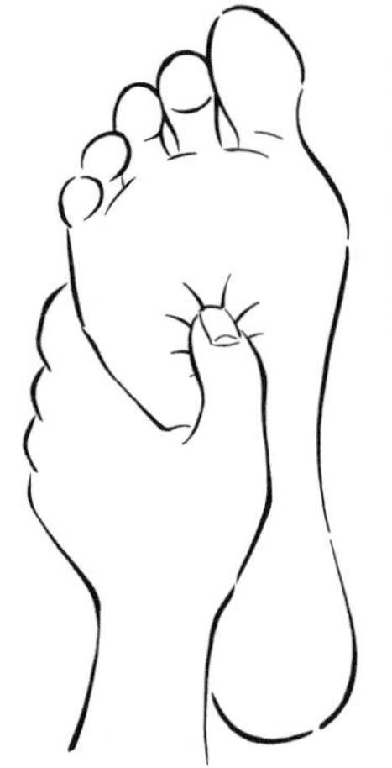

The two pressure techniques for reflexology are (left) pressure on a single spot and (right) rocking the thumb from side to side in a kneading motion.

practice as a reflexologist, so it is sensible to consult a national organization to see if it can recommend an experienced practitioner in your area. Otherwise, try massaging the appropriate areas of your feet. In the case of allergies in general, these are points for the appendix, the adrenals and the ilio-caecum; if you have asthma, concentrate on the points for the lungs and adrenals; if you suffer from hayfever, try massaging the solar plexus point, the points for the adrenals, the lungs and the big toe and the other toes; if you have eczema, massage the points for the kidneys, stomach, liver and spleen.

REFLEXOLOGY POINTS

As a rule, check for any sensitive points by pressing firmly on different areas of the feet and taking note of any tender areas. Make a map of where these points are and work on them.

Knead the points with your thumb (working on tender points on both feet simultaneously, if you have a helper) – but be careful not to dig your thumbnail into the skin. There are two ways of kneading. Try pushing down with the pad of your thumb and at the same time rotating the pressure without moving off the spot for 30 seconds; or move your arm backwards and forwards for 30 seconds, so that the pressure from your thumb is rocked from side to side. Repeat three times on each point.

For hayfever, concentrate on the eye, sinuses and ear reflexology points highlighted in the illustration for about 30 minutes in total, every other day.

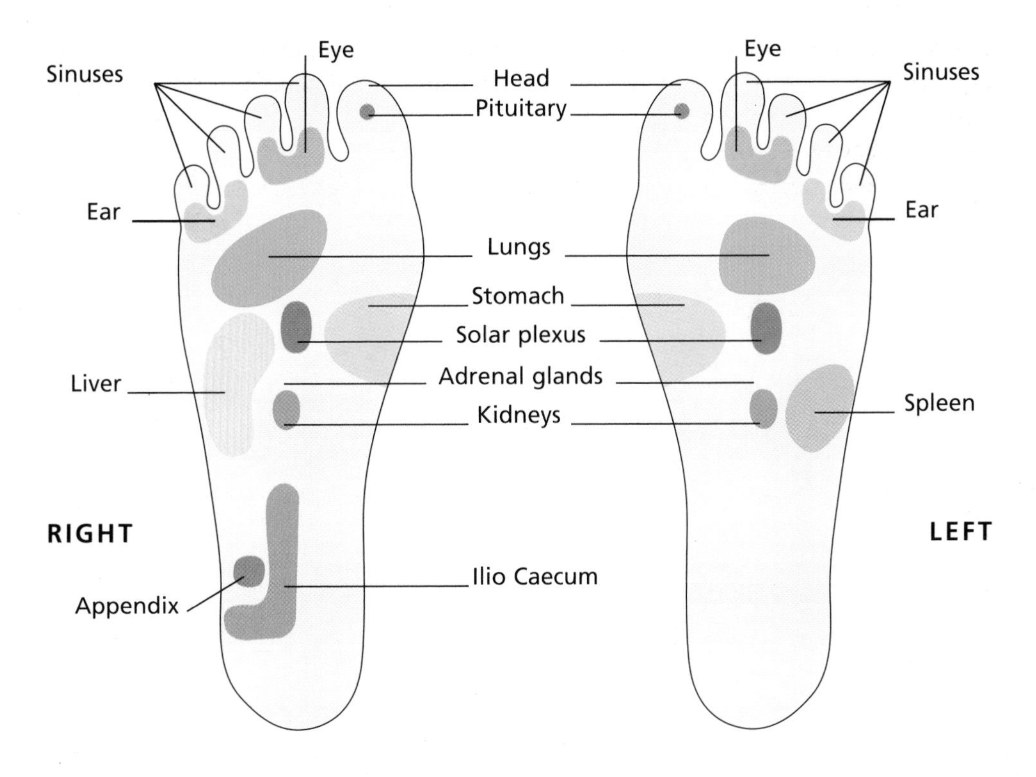

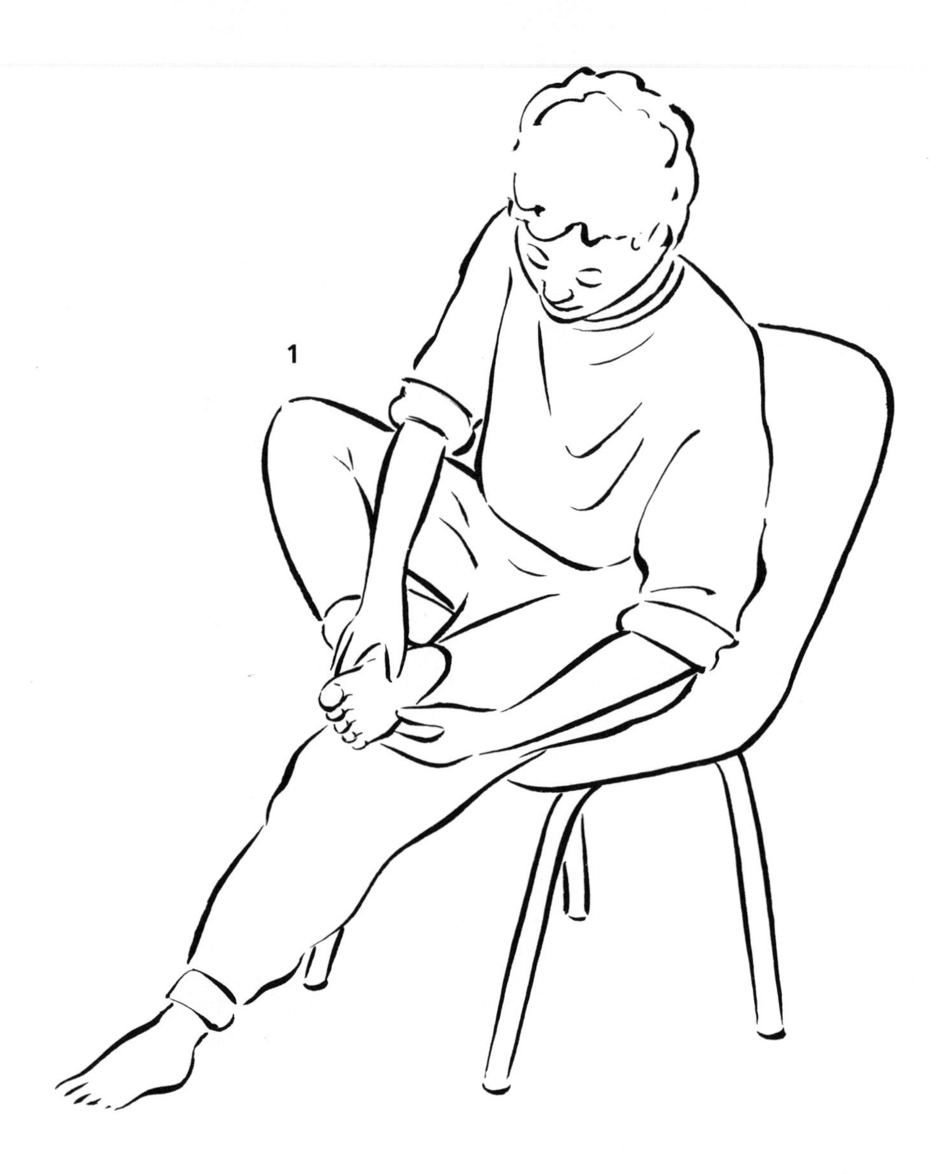

REFLEXOLOGY TECHNIQUES

1 Wash your feet thoroughly in warm water and dry them. Sit in a warm peaceful room with one leg crossed over the other – be careful not to strain your back – so that you can reach the foot with your hands; otherwise, ask a partner to help massage you. Massage your foot thoroughly, using an aromatherapy massage oil (see pp. 82 – 5) or talcum powder, stroking and kneading the flesh, especially on the sole of the foot (**2**).

3 Move all the joints of the foot, starting with the ankle. Circle the ankle with your hands, moving it first in one direction and then the other; move your foot up and down and in and out. Next,

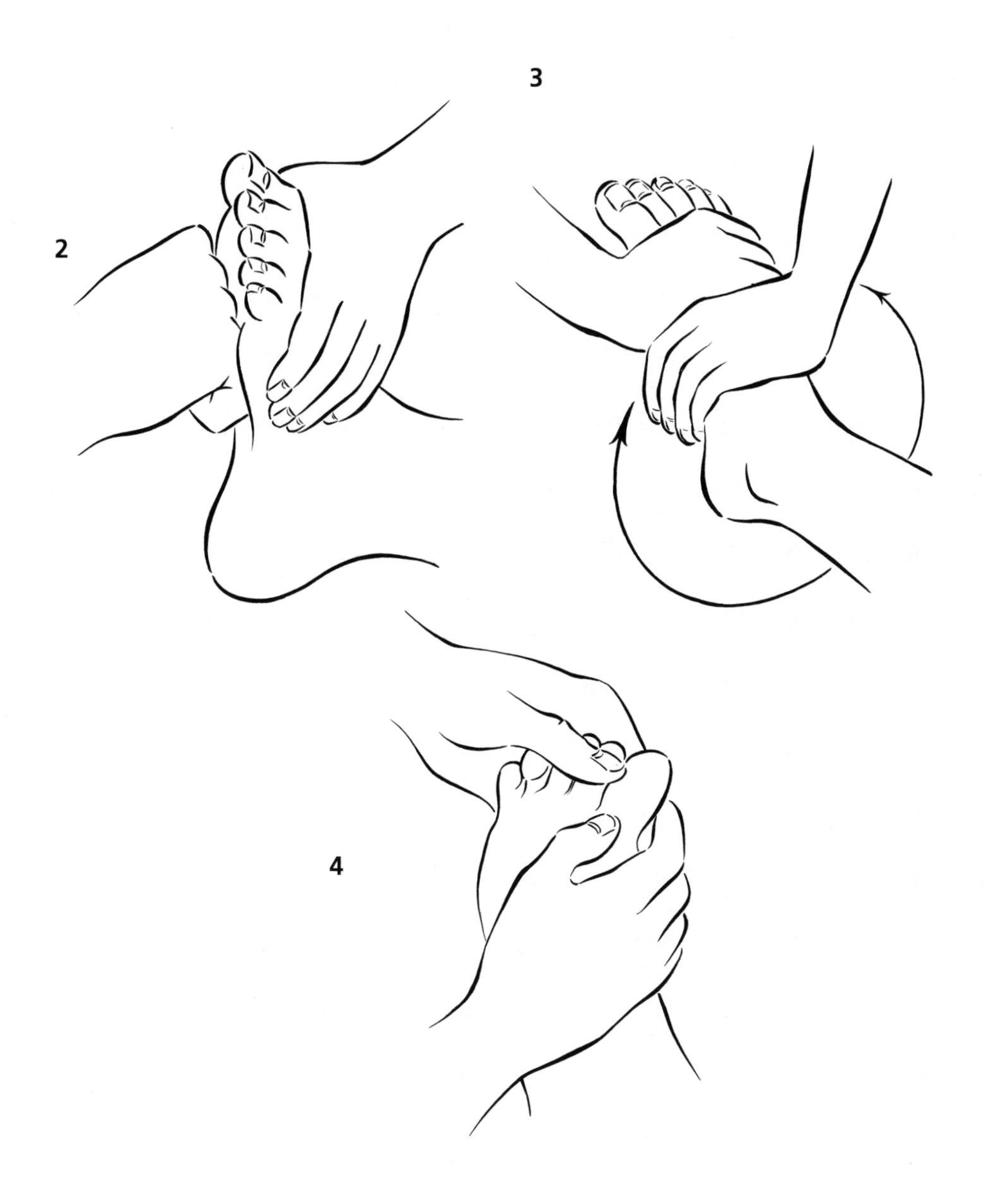

take each toe in turn, starting with the big toe, and bend it first backwards and forwards and then from side to side; then finish by pressing on the pad of each toe and gently pulling the toe as though to lengthen it. Finish with a general massage to the whole foot, then repeat the exercise with the other foot.

4 Once the feet are relaxed, it's time to concentrate on the sensitive reflexology points on the soles of your feet.

Massage and aromatherapy

Massage has a long tradition as a healing therapy and has been used throughout the world for centuries to treat a wide range of disorders and alleviate their symptoms. A truly complementary therapy, massage can help relaxation and improve the quality of rest, and so allow the body's own healing powers to focus on the medical challenges that it faces rather than the problems caused by stress.

Both head and face massages and back and neck massages are effective in achieving this relaxation. Tense, tight upper back and neck muscles, which are often the result of poor posture, can cause headaches, contribute to insomnia and indicate a corresponding over-relaxation in their opposing muscles in the chest – this constricts the airways, which increases the difficulties experienced by allergies that affect breathing, such as hayfever and asthma. A back and neck massage, however, can relax the muscles used for breathing and ease discomfort. And in the case of hayfever, in particular, a face and head massage is not only relaxing but aids the absorption of excess fluids from around the nose and eyes, as well as generally lessening the tightness and irritability of the facial tissues.

The deep relaxation produced by massage also dissipates the harmful effects of the stress (see pp. 12–13) and gives the autonomic system a chance to put itself back into equilibrium, so that the parasympathetic nervous system does not over-react to the presence of allergens and trigger an allergic reaction, with all its associated symptoms.

PREPARATION

Choose a warm, peaceful room and set aside at least half-an-hour for your massage, making sure that there will be no distractions – take your telephone off the hook or switch on your answer machine. Undress from the waist up and remove any necklaces or earrings, then lie on a firm surface – either a bed or the floor – with a pillow covered in a warm towel under your head in the case of a head and face massage or under your lower legs for a back massage. Ask whoever is to give you the massage to wear loose, comfortable clothes and ensure that they have warm hands, and short nails and a bottle of massage oil or a mixture of massage oil and aromatherapy oil (see pp. 86–7) at hand.

Then show them the instructions on this page!

BACK AND NECK MASSAGE

Cover your hands with oil and place them on the body of the person to be massaged – your thumbs should be on either side of the spine below the shoulder blades, and your fingers should point up towards the neck.

1 Stroke firmly up to the top of the neck, across the shoulders and down the back, moulding your hands to the shape of the body. Repeat until the whole area is covered in the oil. Alter the stroke slightly by making circles as you move up the back. Repeat these stroking movements until he or she is relaxed and used to the feel your hands.

2 Starting at the spine at the top of the shoulder blades, use your thumbs to knead the muscles that run up the side of the spine right up to the base of the skull – use small circular movements. (Do not push too firmly at the base of the skull, because this can be dangerous.) Then stroke down again.

3 Taking one side at a time, knead the shoulder muscle from the neck down to the tip of the shoulder. Use both hands and pick the muscle up in your hands. With one hand, squeeze the muscle without pinching; then relax and squeeze with the other hand. This large muscle can hold a great deal of tension and there may be areas that are tender. If so, use your thumbs to push down on the tender spots, rotate slightly without moving off the spot, hold for a few seconds and release. If the pain increases too much, use less pressure. Repeat five times and then move on to another painful spot or continue kneading. Finish the massage with the same stroking movements as at the start.

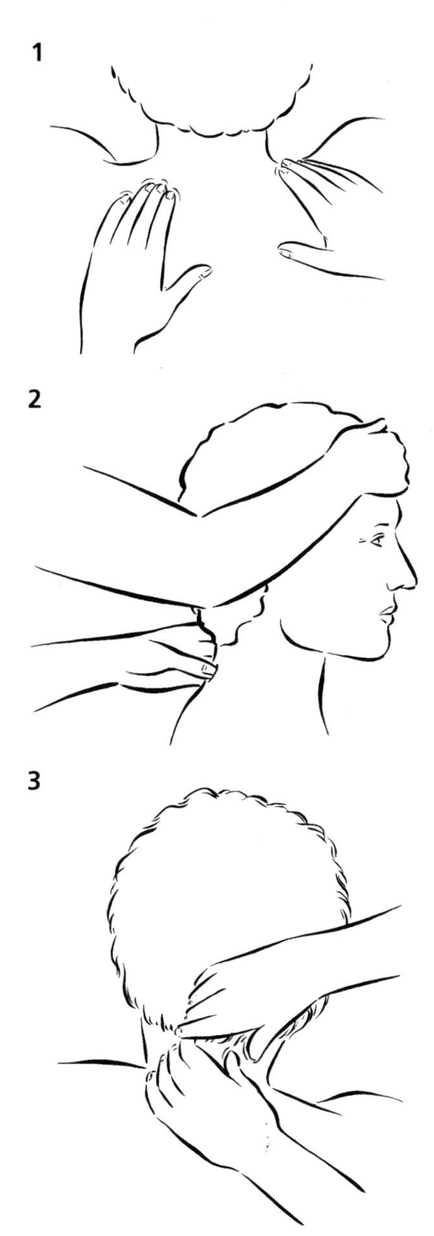

HEAD AND FACE MASSAGE

Lie the person to be massaged on his or her back with the head on a pillow covered with a towel. Stand or kneel behind the head and cover your hands with massage oil – but throughout, be careful not to allow any oil near the eyes.

1 Cup the jaw with your hands and stroke up the sides of the face and across the forehead; pause and press slightly. Then, using only your fingers, gently stroke down each side of the nose and back out across the jaw-line to the dip just in front of the ear above the cheek bone. Pause and press again. Be careful not too pull the skin in any downward movement.

2 With the fingers of each hand, stroke from the chest up the neck to the jaw line.

Using small, circular movements, stroke the cheeks with the pads of your fingers in an upward and outward direction.

3 Place your thumbs at the bridge of the nose and stroke out to the temples. Pause at the hairline and press. Repeat, moving slightly up the forehead each time until you reach the hairline. Continue the stroking movement, but use either your thumbs or fingers in small, circular movements.

Use the pads of your fingers to rub the scalp in circular movements – as though washing the hair thoroughly. You can use scalp oil at this stage, but this will mean that the person being massaged will have to wash his or her hair later, so you may decide not to use any oil at all.

Finish the massage by stroking from the jaw line up to the forehead with your whole hand, pausing over the eyes.

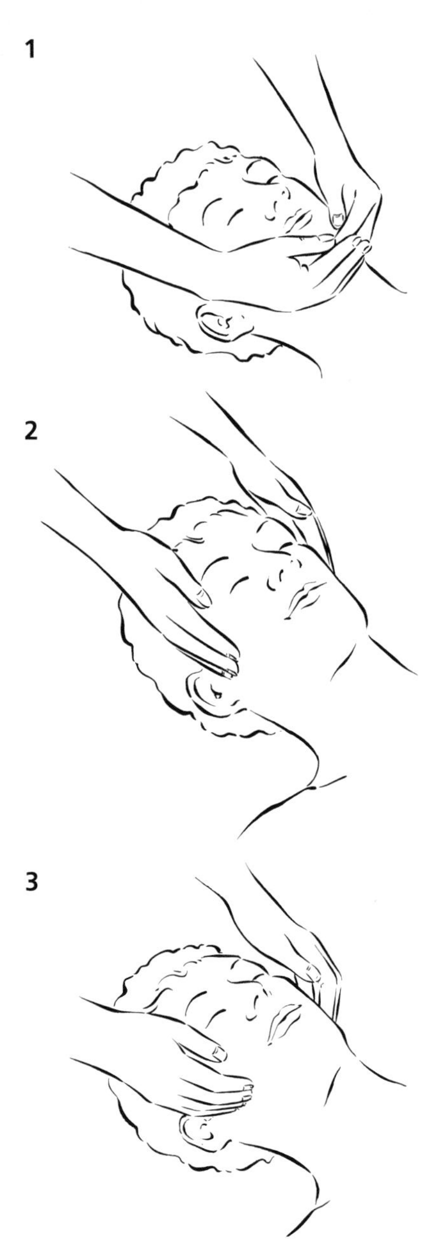

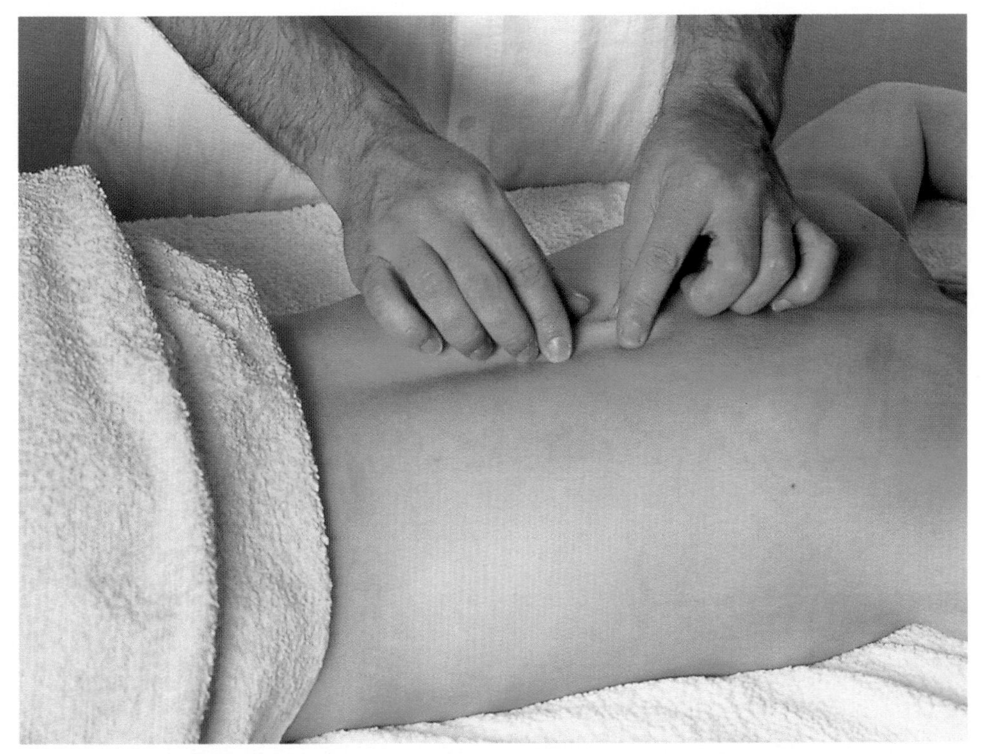

Massage promotes relaxation and a sense of well-being, supporting good health.

USING AROMATHERAPY OILS

Aromatic plants have been used for centuries to perfume people and rooms and to camouflage unpleasant smells. But over the years, healers found that the aromas that are given off by various species of plants have different effects on the psyche – probably because smell is analysed in the same area of the brain as emotions – as well as having unique therapeutic properties. The essential oils used in aromatherapy are harvested from the appropriate flowers, herbs and trees, and used in a variety of ways, such as bathing, inhalation and massage (see pp. 86–7).

Most health stores stock aromatherapy oils. Use a few drops in your bath and inhale the vapours or mix with massage oil, using two drops of aromatherapy oil to 5ml of massage oil (in the case of a head and face massage, use only one drop to 5ml and make sure that the resulting mix is kept well clear of eyes, nostrils and mouth). Make the mixture each time, as stored aromatherapy massage oil goes off fairly quickly.

MEDICAL ALERT

Do not massage anyone who has a high temperature, a skin infection, a contagious disease or a circulatory problem, such as a thrombosis.

Essential oils for allergies

Boswellia thuriferia **(frankincense)**
A deep woody fragrance that lingers with calming and relaxing properties. Make up a massage oil and rub into the chest to relieve congestion in the case of hayfever, or ease the wheeziness of asthma. Try it in the bath as a stress-reliever – it's a wonderful tonic for ageing skin, too!

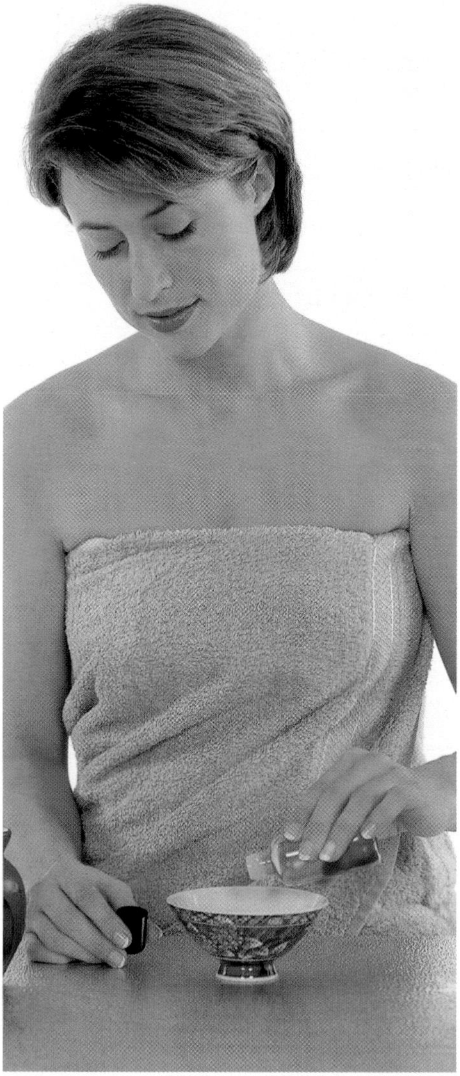

Using essential oils for aromatherapy.

Cedrus libani **(cedarwood)**
A tangy, fragrant oil: use it in the bath to help the relieve mucus congestion and sinusitis of hayfever and the tightness in the chest of mild asthma; or try it in a steam inhalation.

Citrus aurantium **(neroli)**
This oil has a sweet middle note that is very relaxing: use it in the bath to help dry, sensitive or eczematous skin.

Cymbopogon nardus **(citronella)**
A zesty, refreshing oil that helps relieve hayfever symptoms and asthmatic tightness of the chest when used in a steam inhaler. It can also be used to massage the abdomen to help clear up digestive upsets.

Eucalyptus globus **(eucalyptus)**
A fresh, tangy fragrance that works fast but dissipates quickly, it has antiseptic qualities and is very refreshing. Derived from the twigs and the leaves of the fever tree, eucalyptus helps relieve hayfever symptoms when used in a bath and works well as a decongestant when used as a massage oil – try sprinkling a drop on your pillow to help you breathe easily during the night. A few drops in your bath will also help relieve the symptoms of eczema and sensitive skin.

***Illicum anisatum* (aniseed)**
Make up into a massage oil and rub this into the chest and back to relieve hayfever symptoms and asthmatic tightness and wheeziness; it can also be taken as a steam inhalation.

***Lavandula* spp. (lavender)**
The fresh middle note of this oil lifts the spirits and promotes calm and relaxation. Use it in the bath or take advantage of its antiseptic properties by massaging it gently into the area of insect bites.

***Matricaria recutita* (chamomile)**
A fruity, crab-apple smell with a mellow middle note that is calming and soothes the nervous system. It is mildly anti-allergenic, and so is useful if you suffer from eczema or skin sensitivity. Hayfever sufferers find it useful, too, but avoid this is you are allergic to ragweed pollen, because there is a risk of a cross-reaction (see pp. 14–15).

***Melaleuca alternifolia* (tea tree)**
This sharp, spicy oil has germicidal, antiseptic powers, as well as being soothing and healing. Use it in the bath to treat eczema, dry or sensitive skin, insect bites, pimples and boils.

***Pelargonium odorantissimum* (geranium)**
This sharp, tangy, astringent oil is well-known as an insect repellent, but less well-known, perhaps, is that it can be used as to treat insect bites, in a gentle massage. Try it in the bath, too, to combat eczema.

***Rosa* spp. (rose)**
A rich sweet smell that lingers and has anti-inflammatory and mildly sedative properties: try it in the bath to aid relaxation and improve breathing if you suffer from hayfever or asthma.

***Rosmarinus officinalis* (rosemary)**
This oil acts as a mild stimulant to the muscles, so it's ideal as a massage oil for hayfever sufferers and asthmatics – apply to the muscles of the chest and back to ease breathing, relieve congestion and decrease wheeziness.

***Thymus vulgaris* (thyme)**
This herb is all-powerful in the fight against infection, but it's an especially important essential oil when it comes to relieving the tightness and wheeziness of asthma and the congestion of hayfever. Apply to the chest and back in a massage oil, or use in a steam inhaler.

MEDICAL ALERT

Do not use aromatherapy oils if you are pregnant – this is particularly important during the first three months.

Essential oils are highly concentrated and can cause an allergic skin reaction if not correctly diluted.

Essential oils should not be taken internally unless a specialist in internal medicine recommends it – try herbal infusions instead (see pp. 60–65).

Relaxation and exercise

Stress and relaxation are opposite sides of the same coin. We need both to live a rich, varied life and, in the right circumstances, 'good' stress gives us a wonderful rush of adrenaline, heightened awareness, euphoria and excitement. The trouble is that in modern life there is often a lack of balance between the two sides of the coin: with little 'good' stress and equally little relaxation, harmful stress predominates. This is the type of stress that is not dissipated; you hold it inside you, worrying about everything, or carry it around with hunched, tight shoulders as it gnaws away inside you.

As we've seen (see pp. 12–13) this type of stress affects both your mental and physical state and can aggravate a large number of problems as well as actually causing some of them – and allergies are no exceptions to this rule. Asthma and hayfever, in particular, are cases in point, because their mechanism is so closely linked to the stress response; attacks of eczema, too, are known to develop when a sufferer is under stress. And the only way to dissipate the harmful affects of stress is to use up the unspent adrenaline and tension through exercise, or to reduce the amount that is produced by the body by means of relaxation.

What exercise you take and the way in which you prefer to relax are matters of personal taste, and are outside the scope of this book. Nevertheless, it is important that you start some form of exercise – after consulting your doctor, if you are in any doubt about your physical condition – and set yourself a relaxation programme. Many people put off doing so until another day, but that's a mistake, especially as exercise and relaxation can help alleviate the symptoms of an allergic reaction. A 10-minute relaxation routine is given on pp. 90–91 – use it as part of your daily routine – but many other relaxation techniques and therapies are available. Some of them are discussed in this book, such as massage and aromatherapy (see pp. 82–5), self-hypnosis (see pp. 92–3), visualization (see pp. 94–5) and yoga and meditation (see pp. 96–97).

BIOFEEDBACK

It's all too easy to pooh-pooh the importance of relaxation techniques, but their effect has been scientifically proven. What led to the proof was the use of biofeedback techniques, which were first invented in the 1960s, after scientists had built the first machines that could monitor the body's properties, such as the heartbeat (measured by the electrocardiograph, or ECG) and the brain waves (measured by the electroencephalograph, or EEG).

Researchers soon found that people could lower their blood pressure, reduce their pulse rate and change brain waves just by willing them to change while looking at a the results on a monitor. Some people find that they can do even more, such as increasing the number of defensive white cells in the blood (see visualization, pp. 94–5). You can be taught how to will changes in the basic body systems at a biofeedback training centre – many large cities have one – and once the technique has been learned you will soon find that you can put it into practice without the aid of the equipment.

As we have seen (pp. 12–13) the body changes in response to stress hormones, so that when under stress it is in a constant low-level state of the 'fight or flight response' – and these changes involve an increase in blood pressure and muscles tension, among other things. So a system that monitors these factors provides an indicator of your stress levels and degree of relaxation. A variety of machines that do this can be bought for home use, but the easiest of them to use – and it's not expensive – is called a 'relaxometer'. It fits into the palm of one hand while two electrodes are attached to the palm of the other hand; when it is turned on a tone can be heard through earphones. When you are under stress, the tone is high and whining, but as you relax it subsides to a lower-pitched buzz. Use it to monitor not just your stress levels but the success of your relaxation routines. In time, you should acquire the confidence to diagnose your relative levels of stress and relaxation without using the relaxometer. In the meantime, though, you can demonstrate to any sceptics the scientific proof that relaxation techniques work.

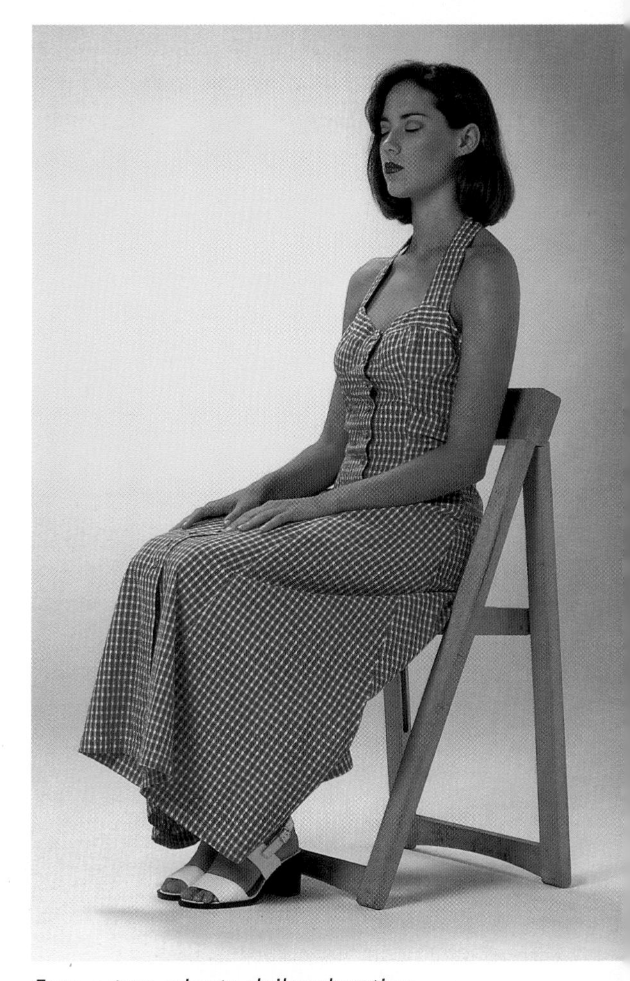

Even a two-minute daily relaxation session will confer positive benefits.

10-minute relaxation

Try to plan ten spare minutes each day for a relaxation routine – and you'll feel the benefit in all areas of your life, as well as improving your chances of avoiding an attack of hayfever. This simple routine contracts and relaxes each of the main muscle groups in turn to release excess muscular tension. It involves tightening each muscle group in turn and then 'letting go'. Each muscle group may need to be tightened and relaxed several times before it 'lets go' of its tension completely.

This routine is the precursor to many more intensive relaxation routines, but if it is performed properly it is still extremely effective. Use it, in whole or in part, anywhere, at any time.

Wear loose, comfortable clothes and lie down on a mat or a bed in a warm peaceful room where you will not be disturbed – take the phone off the hook. Place one pillow under your head and another under your knees and rest your hands, either by your side or on your stomach. Then let your mind go blank and take a couple of deep breaths.

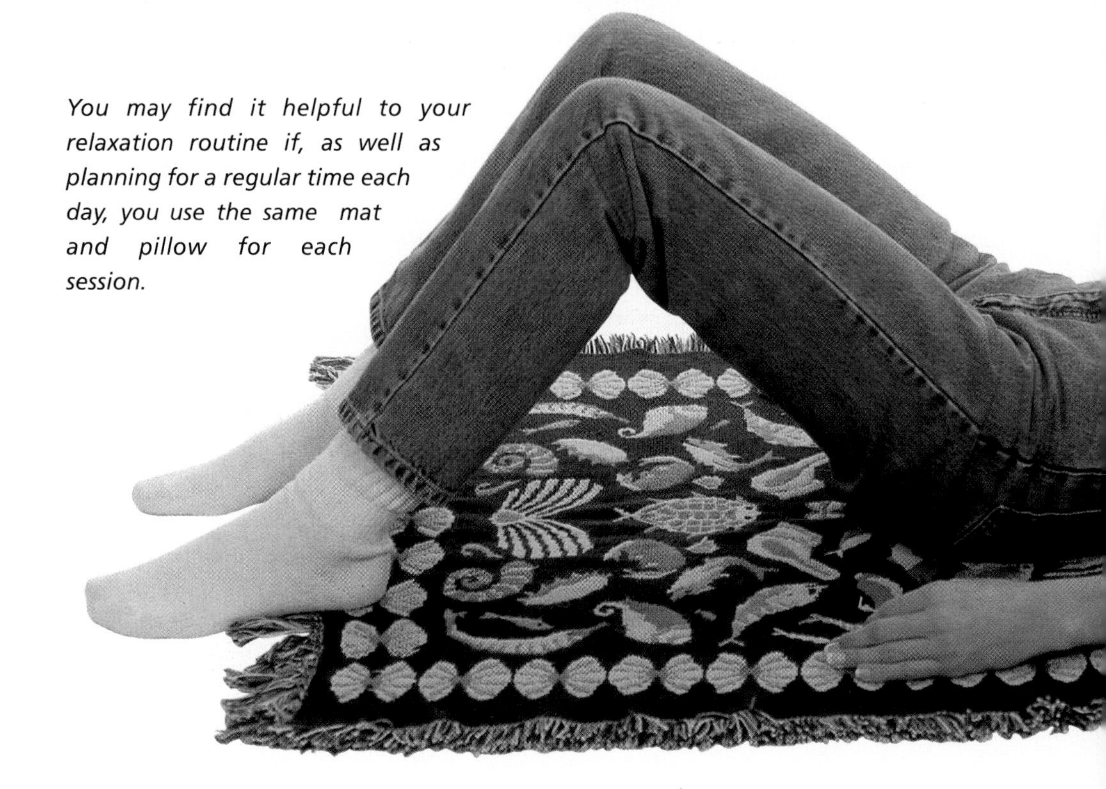

You may find it helpful to your relaxation routine if, as well as planning for a regular time each day, you use the same mat and pillow for each session.

1 Start with your toes: crunch them up tightly, hold and then release. Point your foot down and pull up hard, then release. Circle your ankles in both directions and then crunch up your whole foot and let it go.

2 Move on to your calf muscles, using the same technique, and then up your body to your thigh muscles – you should be able to feel your legs becoming heavier and heavier. If not, tense your whole leg, hold for a few seconds and relax.

3 Move on to your trunk and tighten your abdominal muscles, your buttocks, your back muscles and your chest muscles in turn – feel the tension oozing out of your body.

4 Next, concentrate on your arms. Start with your fingers and taking each part of your arm up to the shoulders – use the same techniques as for your legs. Feel the warmth spread through your body.

5 Hunch your shoulders up towards your ears and release – it may be necessary to repeat this a few times as we all hold a lot of tension in our shoulders, asthma and hayfever sufferers in particular.

6 The head and neck have been left until last because it is sometimes quite difficult to relax them. Rock your head from side to side, then raise your chin to the ceiling. Grimace to relax your face: frown hard, pout your lips, yawn widely and raise your eyebrows, relaxing between each movement.

To finish, tense up your whole body and release then take a few deep breaths. Lie quietly for a couple of minutes before arising refreshed!

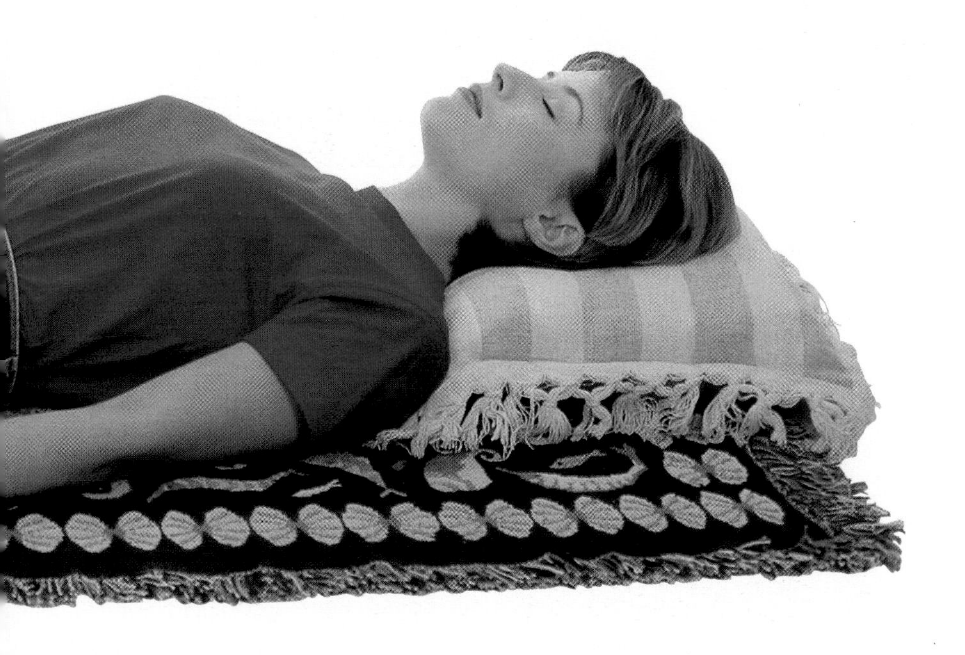

Hypnotherapy

The subconscious mind has a powerful influence on the body – the phrase 'worried sick' can be all too true. Hypnosis is the most direct way of getting in touch with the subconscious mind, and of getting it to work on your behalf. It has been clinically proved to be an effective treatment for asthma, eczema and other forms of allergy. And, once you are used to the technique, self-hypnosis is an easy way to keep your condition under control.

Many people are worried by hypnosis. Stage hypnotism has given the technique a bad name, but in the hands of a reliable, qualified practitioner, hypnosis is a powerful weapon against disease, which has won wide acceptance from the medical profession. It works in two ways. First, it is a form of deep relaxation, with all the benefits that this can bring (see pp. 88–91). Second, it can help to identify and remove any psychological factors that might play a part in your condition. At the same time, it can recruit your subconscious to work on your behalf by implanting positive ideas and images into the mind.

Many people are pleasantly surprised by their first experience of hypnosis. Generally, the therapist will induce only a light trance, in which your muscles become entirely relaxed, and all tension disappears. You will probably feel as if you were sleeping while remaining fully conscious. Many people, after coming round from a hypnotic trance, don't believe they have been hypnotized at all. However, a light trance is quite sufficient for the hypnotherapist to be able to counter irrational fears and to plant beneficial ideas in the mind. Always go to a reputable therapist. Your doctor will probably be able to recommend a suitable practitioner, and there are professional associations which will provide a list of hypnotherapists in your area (see pp. 124 –5).

MEDICAL ALERT

Self-hypnosis should be practised only after consultation with a registered hypnotherapist. You should not try it at all if you have a history of mental disturbance, and you should never implant a potentially dangerous idea.

SELF-HYPNOSIS

Many hypnotherapists will teach you the techniques of self-hypnosis as part of a course of treatment. In fact, the quickest and easiest way of achieving self-hypnosis is through post-hypnotic suggestion. The therapist will plant the suggestion in your mind that you will go into a light trance whenever you perform a particular ritual or set of actions. Once the idea is in your subconscious, simply performing the ritual will put you into a trance in as little as 30 seconds. Commercial tapes are also available but be sure to pick a good one; your therapist may be able to recommend one to you. Eventually, you may want to make a tape of your own, recording the particular positive suggestions and affirmations that you want to hear repeated while you are in a trance.

TIPS FOR SUCCESS

Be convinced about what you are trying to achieve. You cannot persuade your subconscious to do something it really doesn't want to do. Write down the ideas – no more than two or three – you are trying to suggest to your subconscious, and keep the piece of paper with you. Make sure that all statements are positive, not negative. For example, think 'I am breathing easily on a beautiful spring day', not 'I am not suffering from asthma (or hayfever)'.

Use the present tense, and refer to a real situation rather than an intention – the subconscious responds to what is happening here and now, rather than planning for the future. You should say 'I am lying on a sunny beach and my skin is clear and golden', not 'I can go sunbathing and my skin will not itch'.

Tape record the messages you want to send to your subconscious, so that your conscious mind can stay dormant. Finish by recording the routine you use to bring yourself out of a trance.

SIMPLE SELF-HYPNOSIS

Position an object – anything will do – so that you have to look up slightly to see it and focus on it.

Relax completely (see pp. 90–91) and let your mind go blank.

Visualize an up-and-down movement, such as the pendulum of a clock or a see-saw. Watch the movements.

Breathe deeply and feel yourself becoming even more relaxed.

Count down from 10 slowly – try visualizing the lights of a lift going down; as you say each number repeat after it: 'I am sleepy.'

By the time you reach one you should be in a light, relaxed trance but still completely conscious.

Repeat the following phrases before you concentrate on the ideas you want to suggest to your subconscious mind:

'I will wake up completely if there is an emergency.'

'I will stay in this trance no longer than 30 minutes' (or less if you wish) 'and then I will bring myself out of it.'

'I will not slip into a deep trance.'

'I will not go into a trance in a dangerous or inappropriate situation.' (for example when driving).

Then focus your mind on your own suggestions or affirmations. Finally, allow yourself to relax before bringing yourself out of the trance by counting up from one to 10 – by the time you have reached 10 you should be fully awake and feeling refreshed.

Visualization

Imagine yourself on a mossy bank beside a gently flowing stream or, if you prefer, on golden palm-fringed sands beside a warm blue sea. One of the joys of visualisation therapy is that it encourages you to daydream in the most pleasant of fashions. Even ordinary daydreaming helps you to relax and reduces stress. It can be combined with self-hypnosis (see pp. 92–3) and other relaxation techniques (see pp. 88–91) and, when used in an ordered and focused way, it can have strikingly beneficial effects on many allergic conditions, as well as on even more serious diseases, such as cancer.

Like hypnotherapy and meditation, visualization therapy is based on the concept that the subconscious mind has a profound influence on the overall well-being of the body. Visualization harnesses your hidden mental powers to help combat the effects of sickness and disease. It encourages the body's own healing mechanisms to deal more effectively with the causes and symptoms of disease, and helps both mind and body to deal with stress and tension. It is one of the simplest of all self-help techniques, and it is entirely harmless – there are no unpleasant side-effects at all.

The basic technique of visualisation is simple. You are encouraged to create a detailed mental image of what is happening in your body, and to imagine yourself as willing the beneficial forces to win. In the case of allergies, the villains are the mast cells, which produce histamine (see pp. 10–11), which in turn causes the various different symptoms of allergies. Through visualization, you join forces with the beneficial agents that destroy the mast cells or counter their effects.

METHOD

Before you start visualizing the defeat of the mast cells, relax fully (see pp. 88 – 91) and empty your mind of any extraneous thoughts. Settle down in a warm, peaceful room and make sure that you will be undisturbed for at least 15 minutes. Visualization is a very personal therapy, so choose the images that feel right for you and for the form of allergy from which you suffer – obviously images that serve for an asthma sufferer will be different from those that are appropriate for someone with eczema or hives. Remember that the more you understand about your particular condition, the better able you will be to encourage the beneficial forces that are fighting on your behalf.

The important thing is that you are relaxed and comfortable, and able to concentrate on the details of the battle that is going on deep in the tissues of your body. The effects of the therapy can often be enhanced if you take some time to teach yourself a gentle form of self-hypnosis (see pp. 92–3).

Visualize yourself without symptoms. If you have asthma, imagine yourself lying beside a mountain stream: your head is clear; and your breathing is even and deep. If you are a hayfever sufferer, your nose is neither runny nor inflamed and your eyes don't itch: you are lying on a beach (where there is no pollen) or by a waterfall, feeling relaxed and warm.

Visualize your nervous system in action: watch the mast cells vanish from the area of inflammation; imagine your adrenal glands producing more and more anti-histamine and watch it fight the histamine and destroy it.

Visualize your subconscious deciding that it will ignore pollen, house-dust mites or other allergens; tell it that these are harmless and should not be fought.

Once you are able to visualize, you will be able to conjure up the picture whenever you need to do so, and particularly when suffering from an allergic reaction. This ability will help your body fight the over-reaction to allergens and limit the severity of your symptoms.

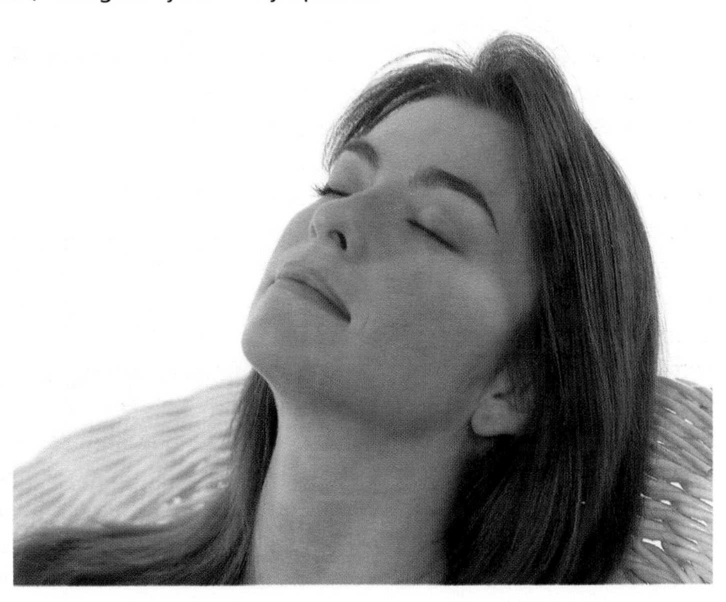

Visualization is a proven self-help strategy in many fields. Even though allergic reactions are real physical conditions, mental focus can help to limit the severity of symptoms and attacks.

MEDICAL ALERT

Take care not to visualize yourself in a situation that involves exposure to your particular allergen or allergens. If you suffer from pollen asthma or hayfever, do not think of yourself in a field full of grass or a summer meadow. If you have a photosensitive form of eczema, do not visualize yourself on a sunny beach. Cases have been reported of allergic attacks being triggered by such visualizations

Meditation and yoga

Yoga and meditation are both derived from ancient Eastern systems of religion and philosophy. Yoga comes from India, where it has been practised for thousands of years, while meditation on its own is an essential part of many Oriental religions. Their primary aim is not so much healing as the restoration of balance and harmony in both body and mind. In many religions, there is an important mystical element in meditation, which is seen as a way of achieving 'oneness' with the universe. However, you do not have to be religious or a philosopher to use these techniques. Their effectiveness has been amply demonstrated, particularly in the case of stress-related allergic conditions.

YOGA

In its Westernized form, yoga has three basic components: postures (Asanas), breathing techniques (Pranayama), and meditation (Dhyana). Yoga should be learned from a qualified teacher – classes are held in most areas (see pp. 124–5) – but once you have mastered the basic techniques, you can easily practise it at home. You don't have to be young or physically fit to take up yoga, but if you suffer from any chronic illness or disability, consult your doctor, and always go to a qualified teacher for advice as to which postures best suit you.

You should set aside at least 20–30 minutes each day for yoga, either first thing in the morning or in the evening. Try to ensure that you will be free from interruption and wear loose comfortable clothes and no shoes. Use an exercise mat if the floor is slippery and keep the room warm to aid relaxation. If you have eaten a heavy meal, wait for three or four hours before practising.

MEDITATION

There are strong similarities between the techniques of meditation and self-hypnosis (see pp. 92–3). Both induce a trance-like state in which the mind is emptied of conscious thought. However, whereas self-hypnosis is used as a way of implanting suggestions into the subconscious mind, meditation has the aim of merging individual consciousness with the greater consciousness of the Cosmos. Even if you are unconvinced by the philosophy, there is no doubt that meditation has brought relief to many people suffering from disease, including those with allergies.

There are many different techniques of meditation, but the most common and widely practised is mantra meditation. In this, the trance-like state is induced by the repetition of a word or words – the mantra. Some people believe that only a guru can choose your mantra for you, but there are plenty of people who have managed perfectly well on their own.

The mantra is usually a word without meaning to you. Such words as 'om' (meaning 'the infinite' in Sanskrit) or 'hum' (meaning 'the infinite within the finite') are widely used. Some teachers have recommended the word 'one', while others have suggested that 'God is love' or simply 'God' can work just as well. You may need to experiment before you find a mantra that is effective for you, but once you have chosen it, you will find that nothing else works quite as well. The technique is simple. Relax in whatever position you have chosen (a yoga posture if so desired) with your eyes closed. Empty your mind of all extraneous thoughts and repeat your mantra over and over again. Your breathing should be steady and regular. If you become aware that you have stopped repeating your mantra, simply start again.

Transcendental meditation is a form of mantra meditation that achieved popularity in the late 1960s and early 1970s, when it was adopted by the Beatles under the guidance of its founder, the Maharishi. It differs from ordinary mantra meditation in that your mantra has to remain a secret and can be given to you only by the guru or an approved teacher. This dependence on the guru has given the movement many aspects of a cult, and there appear to be no increased benefits to be derived from keeping the mantra secret.

Yoga combines mental and physical factors for inner calm.

Two other forms of meditation are 'bubble' (thought) meditation and 'object' (*trataka*) meditation. Bubble meditation differs from other forms of meditation in that thoughts are allowed to enter the mind. You should be relaxed and breathing easily, with your mind emptied. When a thought occurs, regard it passively, as though you were watching it. Picture it as being surrounded by a bubble. As you watch, the bubble slowly rises into the sky until, after about 30 seconds it is lost to sight. Empty your mind again. When the next thought arrives, repeat the process.

In object meditation, you choose a small familiar object – traditionally a candle, but any small object will do – and focus your entire mind on it. The object (or *trataka*) should be a comfortable distance from the eyes, and level with, or slightly below, the eyes. Relax, breathe evenly and concentrate on the object: feel its shape and texture and sense its weight and energy. Allow these sensations to float through your mind. If your concentration lapses, start again.

All types of meditation get easier as you practise them. And all provide the benefits of profound relaxation and the reduction of stress. For best results, each sessionof meditation should go on for at least 15–20 minutes at a time, and should be practised at least once and preferably twice each day.

Alexander Technique

Many people are surprised to learn that posture can have a significant effect on health. They are even more surprised when they discover that posture is involved in every action they take, and that most of the time their posture is poor. The best known posture-correction therapy in the West is the Alexander Technique, named for its Australian founder F.M. Alexander. For allergy sufferers, the technique is most relevant to people with asthma and, to a lesser extent, hayfever, since it can greatly improve breathing. But the sensation of fitness and general well-being that it imparts can benefit allergy sufferers, particularly those whose condition is related to stress.

F.M. Alexander was an Australian actor who found that he had a tendency to lose his voice during a performance. Conventional medicine failed to solve the problem, so he decided to try to find his own solution. He noticed that he had a habit of pulling his head down and in when he was speaking, and he soon discovered that, when he kept his head level, he didn't lose his voice. This led him to make further experiments and observations, and he eventually realized that all our actions involve either good or bad posture – or 'pattern of use' – and that posture can have profound effects on the body, both in mental and physical terms. He began teaching the techniques he had

The Alexander Technique helps the body to learn and maintain good habits of posture.

developed to other actors and singers, and the method gradually spread. The Alexander Technique was born.

We all develop poor postural habits – whether they involve standing, sitting or walking. After a while, these habits feel natural and correct, and any attempt to correct them feels wrong and uncomfortable. For this reason, it is always best to learn the Alexander Technique in classes given by a qualified teacher (see pp. 124–5); after you have mastered the underlying principles, you can practise at home to make your postural modifications permanent.

In fact, continual practice is vital – it takes a considerable amount of effort and time to reject old postural habits and adopt new ones as normal. An Alexander Technique teacher can move with such fluidity that he or she makes everything look easy, but such grace is hard won. You have to become aware of your posture at all times and in all positions, and correct it every time it slips back into former bad habits. But your movements become freer, easier and more economical as you shed the old habitual poor patterns of use and the tensions that they have created are released. In particular, your patterns of breathing will improve, and your general emotional and physical well-being will be increased.

THE TECHNIQUE

Some common postural faults that Alexander Technique teachers look for are those of imbalance – whether one arm hangs further out from the body than the other, for example, or whether the knees roll out when sitting and the back is slouched. They also watch to see if there are unnecessary and unbalanced movements during walking, sitting down and standing up. For example, many people poke their heads back and hunch their shoulders while they are standing up, and then maintain this posture when they are walking rather than straightening up completely. In addition, too long a walking stride entails bracing the knees with each step, which damages the knee joints and puts the spine out of alignment.

Correct posture takes time to learn and to become a natural part of bodily movement.

Once an analysis has been made, the teacher will set out to replace the poor habits with good new ones. This involves the use of hands for physical guidance as well as explanation, example and verbal encouragement. There are no short cuts to postural correction. Actions must be performed many times, under close observation, before the bad habits are finally banished. The first lesson will probably take an hour, and at least six – probably more – further lessons of 30 minutes each will probably be required before the benefits of the technique are fully apparent.

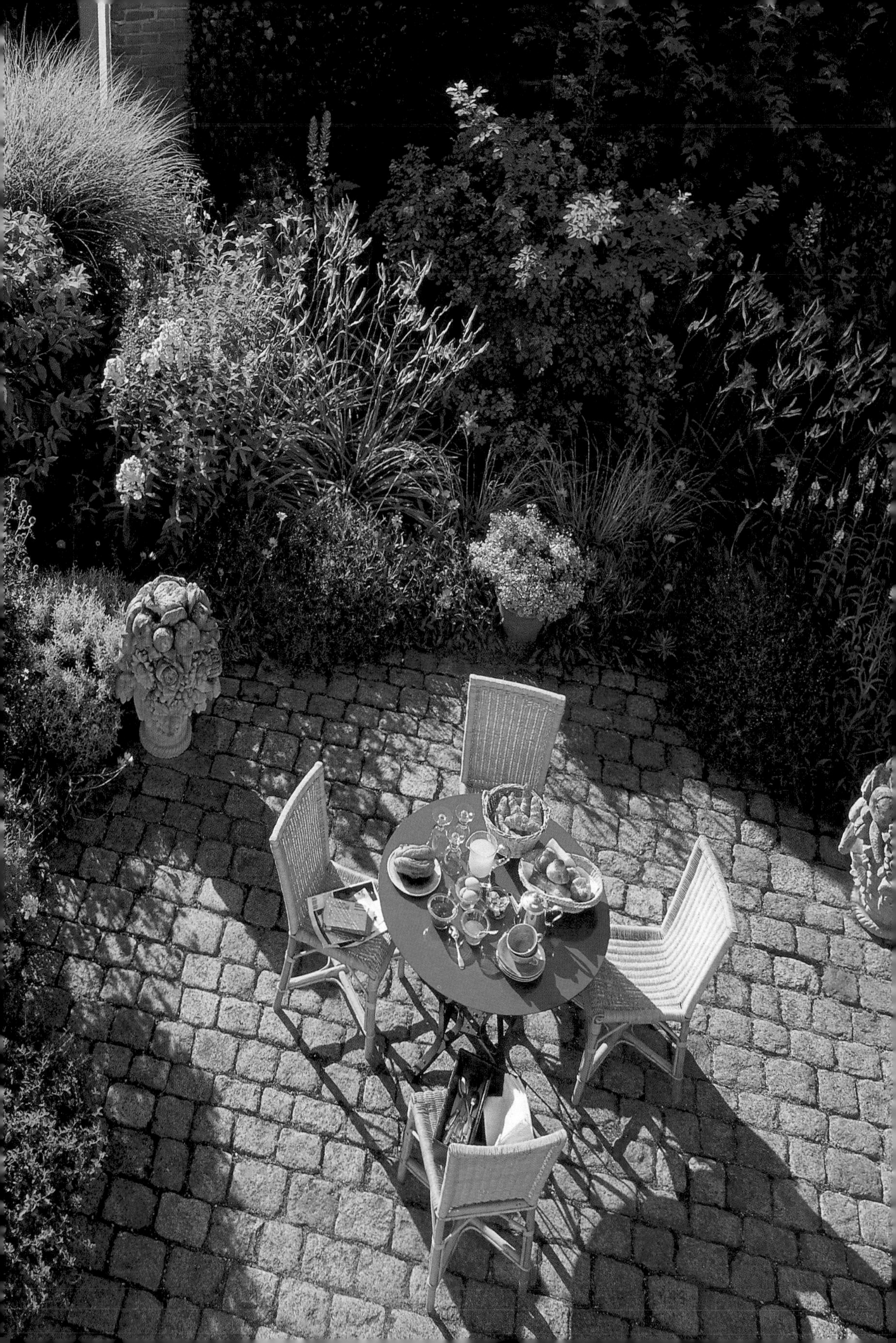

CHAPTER 4

Avoidance and prevention

As an allergic reaction is triggered by a specific substance – or, in the case of asthma, as an attack can be triggered by a specific substance – taking positive steps to avoid that substance will, obviously, reduce the chances of experiencing an allergic reaction. But taking such steps and achieving complete success are easier said than done. As we've seen, something can trigger an attack when it is related, in a biological sense, to the substance to which you are allergic, and all manner of chemicals and food ingredients may lurk, unsuspected, in any product that we buy from our local supermarket. Nevertheless, any avoidance techniques that we practise and preventive measures that we take will help reduce the incidence of allergic responses and improve the quality of life. The following pages outline some of the practical steps that anyone can take to make life with an allergy more bearable.

Know your enemy

Before you can start devising a strategy to avoid a substance to which you are allergic, you have to know what the substance is. That may be stating the obvious, but finding out what causes an allergic reaction can be far from straightforward, because of the very nature of allergies. However, it is possible to devise a structured programme that will enable you to discover what triggers your allergy or, at the very least, that will give doctors a start when they come to test your reaction to specific allergens.

A number of factors complicate the process. First, there is the phenomenon of cross-reactions (see pp. 14–15), which means that materials with chemical or biological similarities to your particular allergen may cause an allergic response. Then there is the problem of masking, which applies particularly in the case of long-term food allergies (see pp. 30–33): the effects of the allergy are obvious, but its cause remains stubbornly difficult to find. And then there is the problem that an allergic symptom can have any one of a large number of causes. Hives, for example, can be triggered by foods, food additives, infections, some drugs, cold, over-exposure to the sun, exercise, stress, certain medical disorders, alcohol, insect bites, tight clothing and the pressure of a car seatbelt.

LOOKING FOR A PATTERN

So how do you find out which of these factors causes your outbreaks of hives, say, or triggers an attack of asthma or hayfever? Sometimes, people with allergies know the answer to this question: if you feel ill and vomit every time you eat shellfish, for example, it's fairly clear that you are allergic to them. But often there is no quick and easy answer to this question. The only way to solve the riddle is to take careful observations of every possible factor that could be linked with the emergence of your symptoms in the hope that a pattern will become apparent – be warned, though, that quite often no pattern will emerge. Nevertheless, the information you record will be invaluable to any doctor who tries to identify the substance to which you are allergic or confirm your identification of it.

TAKING YOUR OWN HISTORY

The first thing to do is to buy a notebook, in which you can record everything about your symptoms, when they affect you and what might have triggered them. At the front of this book, it's well worth recording any family history of allergies, not forgetting the extended family as well as your mother and father. Note down, too, whether you had any childhood allergies – again, record any and all allergies. Next, write down what you can

Hayfever Diary

Month:

DAY/DATE	TIME	POLLEN COUNT	WEATHER	SYMPTOMS	POSSIBLE FACTORS	YOUR ACTIVITIES

remember of any past allergic attacks: How old were you when you first had one? Do you have attacks at particular times of the year? Do you have attacks throughout the year? According to your recollection, did an attack correlate with any particular circumstance?

KEEPING A DIARY

The next step is turn your notebook into a diary of your attacks. We have already discussed how to try to identify a food allergy by means of a food diary and an elimination diet (see pp. 56–7), and the same principle applies here – though it must be extended to all areas of life. Each time you suffer from the symptoms of an allergy you should record the following information:

- the time of day
- the day and month
- any food or drink that you have taken
- if you suffer from hayfever or asthma, the outside pollen count; ring a pollen line to check this (see pp. 124–5)
- the weather, including notes on the approximate temperature and whether it was was it dry, humid, windy or wet
- a note of the symptoms and how long the attack lasted: How long were your eyes and nose running? Was there any wheeziness or tightness in the chest? Were there any skin symptoms? Did you vomit or have diarrhoea? Did you have a headache?
- any associative factors: Had you been in a room with a cat or dog? Had you been outside during harvest-time? had you been walking near busy traffic? Had you been taking exercise?
- What had you been doing in the hour or so before the attack started?

It will take several weeks, if not months, before you can start to draw any tentative conclusions from an analysis of this diary – in fact, in some circumstances it may take a whole year for any positive result to emerge. It may well be worth keeping a diary up, though, because if you take action on the basis of what it reveals, especially if your conclusions are confirmed by a skin test (see pp. 104–105), you may be able to avoid the problem.

For example, after cutting the grass with a petrol motor mower you note hayfever symptoms, plus wheeziness. Was grass pollen the cause? Or was it the sandwich you ate when you took a break? There is also a possibility that there is a cross-reaction with exhaust fumes from the mower. Wheeziness and tightness in the chest after exercise may indicate that there is a tendency to asthma, which may be triggered equally by the pollen, the exhaust fumes or exercise. However, this diagnosis is only provisional, and many other possibilities need to be ruled out before any definite conclusions can be drawn. It is important that you do not take any action without consulting your doctor.

READING THE SIGNS

When you have a reasonable amount of data, it's time to see if you can reach any conclusions. Is there any repeated association between something you do, somewhere you go or something you eat and drink and your symptoms? It's often possible to draw some preliminary conclusions. If, for example, you are an asthmatic and your asthma attacks are mainly confined to the late summer, autumn and early winter, it's likely that your problem is caused by house-dust mites; on the other hand, spring and summer attacks that recur, though with lesser severity, into the autumn, could well be caused by a pollen allergy that also makes you sensitive to mite droppings. If your attacks are seasonal, but out of step with pollen counts, they may be triggered by an allergy to the spores of a particular mould – to which one can be indicated by a match with the season for that mould and confirmed by a skin test.

In the case of pure pollen allergies, however, things are a little more simple, because you can cross-reference the pattern of your symptoms directly to pollen seasons (see pp. 108–115). You can then confirm your suspicions by use of avoidance and prevention techniques, and you will know if you are correct and will be able to set a pattern of living for the future if they are successful at reducing the number and severity of attacks.

It is important that you do not attempt to act on any suspicions yourself: consult your doctor before taking any action, because there is always a risk that you will make a mistake and make your condition worse – dangerously so. But even if no firm conclusions come to mind when you examine your diary, a specialist may be able to derive useful information from it, so take it to any consultation.

CONFIRMING YOUR SUSPICIONS

Your diary may well lead you to suspect the identity of the substance to which you are allergic, or at least the family to which it belongs, but confirmation of its precise nature can come only from the results of a skin test. There are four different types of skin test – a scratch test, a skin prick test, an injection and a patch test – but all rely on the same principle: a series of different allergens are put in contact with the tissues to see which one causes an allergic reaction.

Scratch tests and skin prick tests are the ones most often used by allergists. Both are easy to administer and virtually pain-free. They also have the advantage that as many as 30 different tests can be carried out at the same consultation.

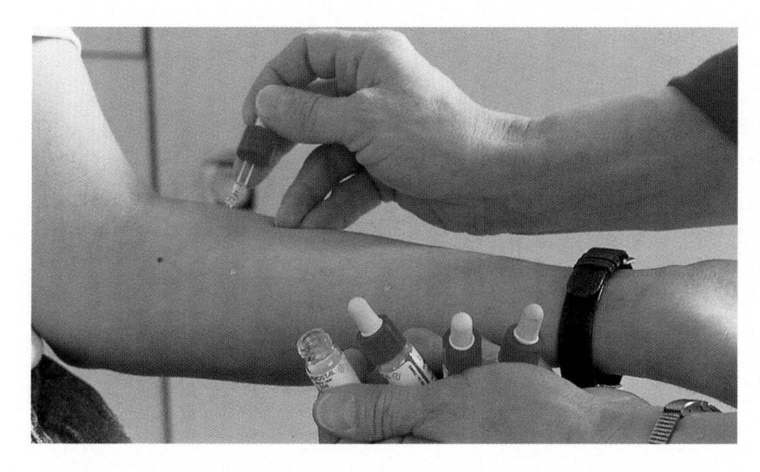

A skin prick test in progress. Drops of allergens in liquid form are applied to pricked areas of the patient's arm. Any inflammation indicates a possible allergy to that particular substance.

In the case of a scratch test, the skin is scraped with a needle and a sample of a particular allergen is dropped onto the scratch: if you are sensitive to that allergen, the area of the scratch will become red and swollen – the larger and redder the bump, the greater the sensitivity. In skin prick tests, the allergen is dropped onto the skin, which is then pierced with a needle or lancet in order that the allergen can come into direct contact with the mast cells in the tissues. The response is positive if the site becomes red, swollen and itchy.

Sometimes, an allergist may inject a series of allergens into the superficial layers of the skin at intervals of about 2.5cm (1inch). This is the most accurate of the various types of skin test, but it is usually only performed if there is a definite suspicion of what the allergen might be – this is where your diary comes in handy. A generalized, non-specific reaction to the allergen is ruled out by administering a highly diluted dose first. Again, a redness and soreness indicates that you are allergic to that particular allergen.

A patch test works on the same principles as the other tests, but in this case the skin is not ruptured at all. The allergen is placed on a piece of soft cloth or paper and stuck on the skin by a plaster, which stays in place for 48 hours before being removed. Any reaction at the site indicates a sensitivity to the allergen. This test is occasionally used in cases of hayfever, but its primary purpose is to test skin allergies to metals and chemicals.

MEDICAL ALERT

A positive reaction to an allergen is normally confined to the site of the test, but in rare cases, when the subject is extremely allergic to a substance, the test may trigger more generalised symptoms such as wheezing, general itching, hives and sneezing. And in exceptional cases a skin test can trigger an asthma attack or even lead to anaphylactic shock (see pp. 24–5). For this reason it is important that you consult a qualified allergist who has resuscitation equipment on hand.

Avoiding food and drug allergies

Even if you know what you are allergic to, it is not always easy to avoid it. Fortunately, the contents ofmost foods and over-the-counter drugs are clearly shown on the packaging, so that, provided you check the labels carefully, you can avoid those that contain your particular allergen. When you buy a prescription drug, always ask your doctor or pharmacist to check the product information to ensure that it doesn't contain an additive , such as a colouring agent, to which you may be allergic

FOOD FAMILIES

An allergy to one particular type of food is often accompanied by an allergy to other members of the same food family. Below are listed some common allergens, as well as the foods to which they are related and that might also trigger an allergic reaction.

- Apple, pear quince
- Artichoke, chicory, endive, lettuce, sunflower, tarragon
- Buckwheat, rhubarb, sorrel
- Cashew nuts, mango, pistachio nuts
- Grapefruit, kumquat, lemon, lime, tangerine
- Cardamom, ginger, turmeric
- Barley, cane, corn, millet, oats, rice, rye, sorghum, wheat, wild rice
- Avocado, bay leaves, cinnamon, sassafrass
- Asparagus, chives, garlic, leeks, onion, sarsparilla
- Melons, courgettes, cucumber, marrow, pumpkin
- Mint, basil, rosemary, sage
- Bilberry, currants, gooseberry, mulberry
- Broccoli, brussels sprouts, cabbage, cauliflower, horseradish, kale, mustard, radish, swede, turnip, watercress
- Aniseed, caraway seed, carrot, celery, coriander, cumin, dill, fennel, parsley, parsnip
- Acacia, black-eyed peas, licorice, lima beans, peanuts, peas, pinto beans, string beans
- Almond, apricot, cherry, nectarine, peach, plum
- Aubergine, bell peppers, cayenne, chilli peppers, paprika, potato, tomato
- Blackberry, boysenberry, loganberry, raspberry, strawberry
- Poultry and their eggs
- Crabs, crayfish, lobster, prawns, shrimps, squid
- Cows, goats, pigs, sheep and their meat, by-products and milk
- Abalone, clams, mussels, oysters, scallops

FOOD ADDITIVES

While almost any food additive can cause an allergic reaction, those most often implicated are listed here:

E102	Tartrazine
107	Yellow 2G
E110	Sunset yellow FCF *(Orange yellow S)*
E122	Carmoisine *(Azorabine)*
E123	Amaranth
E124	Ponceau 4R *(Cochineal red A)*
128	Red 2G
E151	Black PN *(Brilliant black BN)*
154	Brown FK
155	Brown HT *(Chocolate brown HT)*
E180	Pigment rubine *(Lithol rubine BK)*

Also to be avoided by allergy sufferers are the coal tar dyes:

E104	Quinoline yellow
E127	Erythosine BS
E131	Patent blue V
E132	Indigo carmine *(Indigotine)*
133	Brilliant blue FCF

In addition, certain chemical additives used as preservatives are known to cause problems. These include:

Benzoates	E210-E219
Sulphur dioxide and sulphites	E220-E227
Nitrites and nitrates	E249-E252
Antioxidants	E320,E321

Certain additives have also been shown to have adverse effects on asthma sufferers and people with aspirin allergy. These are:

Benzoates	E210-E219
Gallates	E310-E312
Monosodium glutamate and its relatives	E621-E623 E627, E631, E635

AVOIDING ASPIRIN SENSITIVITY

The active ingredient of aspirin is salicylic acid, and many people who are sensitive to aspirin are also sensitive to a wide range of foods and drinks which contain natural salicylate. A low-salicylate diet may therefore benefit anyone who has had aspirin-sensitive asthma or aspirin-induced hives. Foods with a high natural salicylate content include:

Fruits and nuts – Almonds, apples, apricots, avocados, berry fruits of all kinds, brazil nuts, cherries, coconut, currants, dates, figs, gooseberries, grapefruit, grapes, guavas, lemons, lychees, macadamia nuts, mandarins, nectarines, oranges, passion fruit, peaches, peanuts, pears (unpeeled), persimmons, pineapples, pine nuts, pistachio nuts, plums, prunes, quinces, raisins, rhubarb, sesame seeds, walnuts, waterchestnuts

Vegetables – Asparagus, aubergines, beetroot, broad beans, broccoli, carrots, chicory, chilli peppers, courgettes, cucumber, endive, green beans, marrow, mushrooms, okra, olives, onions, parsnips, bell peppers, potatoes (unpeeled), radishes, spinach, sweetcorn, sweet potatoes, tomatoes, turnips, watercress

Herbs and spices – Many of these have high salicylate levels

Drinks – Coffee, tea, cola, and most fruit juices and alcoholic drinks

Other – Honey, licorice and peppermint tea contain appreciable amounts of salicylate, as do some toothpastes, chewing gums, lozenges, mouthwashes, antiseptics and cosmetics

Foods low in salicylates include all meats, fish, including shellfish, dairy products and eggs. Gin and vodka are among the few alcoholic drinks to have a low salicylate content.

Avoiding pollen

If you suffer from hayfever or you are an asthmatic whose attacks can be triggered by pollen, you are at risk only at certain times of the year. As a result, a large proportion of the year is likely to be trouble-free – if, that is, you also take preventive measures to banish other allergens that might also trigger an attack from your home, such as house-dust mites and animal proteins (see pp. 116–19).

The trouble is that different types of pollen becomes airborne at different times of the year – and the time of year varies according to where in the world you are, which is an important factor to take into consideration when planning a holiday or a business trip. Use the charts on the following pages to determine when the pollen to which you are allergic – which may trigger hayfever or an asthma attack – is likely to be in the air, not forgetting to make a note of when other pollens in the same biological family appear, because these may cause a cross-reaction (see pp. 14–15).

But what should you do at these times? The answer is to stay at home if you possibly can and take the appropriate precautions (see pp. 116–19). Of course, most of us have work to do, so we have to go outdoors. But you can still try to plan your day if you bear in mind a few basic strategies. First, you should ring one of the pollen lines (see pp. 124–5) every day during the season for your pollen to see what local conditions are. This is because the time of day that pollen is most likely to be present in the air varies according to local conditions, and in particular according to the local weather in the geographical area where you live.

For example, in general plants release pollen early in the morning, but the time varies according to the species. Ragweed, for example, tends to release pollen from around dawn to 9am, while grass pollen is released from about 7.30am to 10am (although some grasses release pollen later in the day). But if conditions are damp and cold, the pollen will not leave the flower; and if it is raining, the pollen will be washed away, so you are unlikely to have any problem. If the weather is mild and there is a light breeze, however, the pollen will be blown around in the air and an allergic response is a distinct possibility.

The trouble is that things are not that simple. On a warm, sunny day, for example, the morning sun will warm up the air, and it will rise into the atmosphere, taking the pollen with it. The pollen will stay high in the atmosphere until the air cools, either because the sun has set or the weather has changed. But when the air has cooled, the pollen will fall back to ground. This means that pollen may not begin to fall and give rise to an attack of hayfever or asthma until a few hours after sunset – or later than this if you live in a city, where the ground air stays warmer for longer.

An added complication is the phenomenon known as 'inversion'. If you live in a valley or low-lying area that is surrounded by high ground, a layer of cold air is likely to hug the ground, even though there may be warmer air above it. The result is that the air at ground level does not rise, and all the pollen is trapped near the ground, together with any other pollutants that there might be, giving a high risk of hayfever and asthma.

To sum up: the main danger comes when a warm, dry day follows a period of cold and dampness, which will have caused build-up of pollen in the plants. You should take precautions against exposure to pollen in the late evening if you live in the country, or from the late evening to late at night if you live in a city. But if you live in a valley or low-lying area surrounded by high ground, you may be at risk all day long.

POLLEN SEASONS ROUND THE WORLD

Hayfever sufferers planning a trip need to know the times to avoid if possible. The chart below and on the pages following summarizes information from around the world. Peak pollen seasons are given for trees (T), weeds (W), shrubs (S), grasses (G) and farm crops (C).

GREAT BRITAIN AND IRELAND

MONTH		PLANT NAME
February-March	T	*Ulmus* (elm)
February-April	T	*Alnus* (alder)
	T	*Carpinus* (hornbeam)
	T	*Corylus* (hazel)
March-May	T	*Populus* (poplar)
	T	*Salix* (willow)
April-May	S	*Myrica gale* (bog myrtle)
	T	*Acer* (maple and sycamore)
	T	*Aesculus* (horse chestnut)
	T	*Betula* (birches)
	T	*Fagus* (beech)
	T	*Fraxinus* (ash)
	T	*Pineaceae* (pine)
	T	*Platanus* (plane)
	T	*Quercus* (oak)
April-September	W	*Asteraceae* (dandelion)
	W	*Compositae* (goldenrod)
May-June	T	*Juglans* (walnut)
	S	*Ligustrum* (privet)
May-July	S	*Sambucus* (elder)
	W	*Rumex* (dock and sorrel)
	G	*Gramineae*
	G	*Poaceae*
May-October	W	*Amaranthaceae* (amaranth)
	W	*Chenopodiaceae* (goosefoot)
June-July	T	*Castanea* (chestnut)
June-September	W	*Parietaria* (pellitory-of-the-wall)
	W	*Ambrosia* (ragweed)
	W	*Urtica* (nettle)
July-September	S	*Erica, Calluna* (heathers)
	C	Oil-seed rape
	W	*Artemisia* (mugwort, wormwood)

SCANDINAVIA

This area includes Finland, Sweden, Norway and Denmark.

MONTH		PLANT NAME
March-May	T	*Ulmus* (elms)
April-May	T	*Alnus* (alder)
	T	*Corylus* (hazel)
	T	*Myrica gale* (bog myrtle or sweet gale)
April-June	T	*Betula* (birches)
May	T	*Fraxinus* (ash trees)
May-June	T	*Quercus* (oaks)
May-July	T	*Pinaceae* (pines)
	T	*Cupressaceae* (cypresses)
May-August	G	*Gramineae*
	G	*Poaceae*
June-August	T	*Plantagago* (plantains)
	W	*Rumex* (docks)
	W	*Urtica* (nettles)
July-September	S	*Artemisia* (mugwort and wormwoods)

ACKNOWLEDGEMENTS

In preparing this chart, the publisher would like to acknowledge information published by Dr Jean Emberlin of the Pollen Research Unit at the University of North London, Professor Eugenio Dominguez-Vilches of the University of Cordoba, and Professor Walter H. Lewis and Dr Prathiba Vinay of Washington University.

NORTHERN AND EASTERN EUROPE

This area includes Austria, Belgium, Czechoslovakia, northern France, Germany, Hungary, Luxembourg, the Netherlands, Poland and Switzerland.

MONTH		PLANT NAME
February-May	T	*Alnus* (alder)
	T	*Carpinus* (hornbeam)
	T	*Corylus* (hazel)
	T	*Cupressaceae* (cypresses)
March-April	T	*Taxus* (yew)
March-May	T	*Platanus* (plane trees)
April-May	T	*Betula* (birches)
	T	*Fraxinus* (ash trees)
April-June	T	*Fagus* (beeches)
	T	*Quercus* (oaks)
April-July	T	*Pinaceae* (pines)
April-September	G	*Gramineae*
	G	*Poaceae*
May-August	W	*Rumex* (docks and sorrels)
May-September	W	*Pellitories* (parietaria)
	T	*Plantagago* (plantains)
May-October	W	*Amaranthaceae* (amaranths)
	W	*Henopodiaceae* (goosefoots)
June-July	T	*Castanea* (chestnut trees)
June-September	W	*Urtica* (nettles)
July-September	S	*Artemisia* (mugwort and wormwoods)
August-September	W	*Ambrosia* (ragweeds)

SPAIN & PORTUGAL

MONTH		PLANT NAME
January-March	T	*Cupressaceae* (cypresses)
February-March	T	*Alnus* (alder)
February-May	T	*Fraxinus* (ash trees)
March, April or May	T	*Platanus* (plane trees)
March-June	T	*Plantago* (plantains)
	T	*Quercus* (oaks)
March-July	T	*Pinaceae* (pines)
March-May or May-July	W	*Pellitories* (parietaria)
April	T	*Betula* (birches)
April-June	G	*Gramineae*
		Poaceae
May-June	T	*Olea* (olive trees)
	T	*Eucalyptus* (eucalyptus or gum trees)
May-July	W	*Urtica* (nettles)
May-September	W	*Amaranthaceae* (amaranths)
	W	*Chenopodiaceae* (goosefoots)
June-August	C	*Helianthus* (sunflowers)
August-September	S	*Artemisia* (mugwort and wormwoods)
October-November	T	*Casuarina* (she-oaks or 'Australian pines')

THE MEDITERRANEAN

This area covers southern France, Greece, Italy and the Mediterranean islands. (The information supplied for Turkey and the Balkans may be more applicable for northeastern Greece.)

MONTH		PLANT NAME
January-May	T	*Alnus* (alder)
	T	*Corylus* (hazel)
February-May	T	*Acacia* (mimosa)
March-April	T	*Populus* (poplars)
March-July	T	*Olea* (olive trees)
	T	*Pinaceae* (pines)
	W	*Parietaria* (pellitories)
April-May	T	*Betula* (birches)
	T	*Broussonetia papyrifera* (paper mulberry)
April-June	T	*Quercus* (oaks)
	W	*Urtica* (nettles)
April-September	G	*Gramineae*
		Poaceae
	W	*Rumex* (docks and sorrel)
May-September	T	*Plantago* (plantains)
May-October	W	*Amaranthaceae* (amaranths)
	W	*Chenopodiaceae* (goosefoots)
June-July	T	*Castanea* (chestnuts)
August-September	W	*Ambrosia* (ragweeds)
August-October	S	*Artemisia* (mugwort and wormwoods)
September-November	W	*Parietaria* (pellitories)
December-June	T	*Cupressaceae* (cypresses)

THE CANARY ISLANDS

MONTH		PLANT NAME
April	G	Grasses

TURKEY AND THE BALKANS

This area includes Bulgaria, Romania, Turkey and the countries of the former Yugoslavia.

MONTH		PLANT NAME
February-May	T	*Alnus* (alder)
	T	*Carpinus* (hornbeam)
	T	*Corylus* (hazel)
	T	*Ostrya* (hop-hornbeam)
March-April	T	*Populus* (poplars)
	T	*Fraxinus* (ash trees)
March-May	T	*Acer negundo* (box elder or ash-leaved maple)
	T	*Cupressaceae* (cypresses)
March-August	W	*Urtica* (nettles)
April-May	T	*Betula* (birches)
	T	*Fagus* (beeches)
	T	*Platanus* (plane trees)
April-May	T	*Quercus* (oaks)
	T	*Erica arborea* (tree heather)
April-June	W	*Rumex* (docks and sorrels)
April-July	T	*Pinaceae* (pines)
May-June	T	*Olea* (olive trees)
May-August	T	*Plantago* (plantains)
	W	*Pellitories* (parietaria)
May-September	G	*Gramineae*
	G	*Poaceae*
June-October	W	*Amaranthaceae* (amaranths)
	W	*Chenopodiaceae* (goosefoots)
July-September	S	*Artemisia* (mugwort and wormwoods)
August-September	W	*Ambrosia* (ragweeds)
September-October	T	*Erica arborea* (tree heather)

THE FORMER USSR

In Russia (west of the Urals), Belarus, the Ukraine and the Caucasus region, the pollen seasons are similar to eastern Europe (see above). No information regarding the other countries in this region.

THE MIDDLE EAST

Lebanon, and western Jordan and Syria.

MONTH		PLANT NAME
March-May	G	Grasses
May-June	T	*Olea* (olive trees)
August-October	S	*Artemisia* (mugwort)

ISRAEL

MONTH		PLANT NAME
March-June	G	Grasses
May-June	T	*Olea* (olive trees)

IRAN

MONTH		PLANT NAME
November-February	T	*Cupressaceae* (cypresses)

EGYPT (ALEXANDRIA REGION)

MONTH		PLANT NAME
mid-February-early December	G	Grasses
late February-November	W	*Chenopodiaceae* (goosefoot)
	W	*Urtica* (nettles)

INDIA & PAKISTAN

Except for the far south, February-April will have the lowest pollen counts. Some level of pollen throughout the remaining months.

NORTH AFRICA

The northern coast of Morocco, Algeria and Tunisia.

MONTH		PLANT NAME
March-May	G	Grasses
May	T	*Olea* (olive trees)

WEST AFRICA

The savanna region from the rainforests north to the Sahel, Nigeria and northern Ghana.

MONTH		PLANT NAME
April-November	G	Grasses

EAST AFRICA – KENYA

MONTH		PLANT NAME
September-October,	G	Grasses
December-January	G	Grasses

EAST AFRICA – THE SAVANNAS OF TANZANIA

MONTH		PLANT NAME
June-December	G	Grasses

EAST AFRICA – ZIMBABWEE

MONTH		PLANT NAME
all year round but peaking in July-August, October-November	G	Grasses

EAST AFRICA – MALAWI

MONTH		PLANT NAME
October-February	G	Grasses

SOUTHERN AFRICA – BOTSWANA

MONTH		PLANT NAME
November-April	G	Grasses

SOUTH AFRICA

Most months of the year peaking:

SOUTH AFRICA – CAPE TOWN

MONTH		PLANT NAME
November-January	G	Grasses

SOUTH AFRICA – JOHANNESBURG AND PRETORIA

MONTH		PLANT NAME
December-January	G	Grasses

JAPAN

MONTH		PLANT NAME
February-April	T	*Cryptomeria japonica* (Japanese red cedar)
February-May	T	*Betula* (birches)
March-April	T	*Alnus* (alders)
	T	*Cupressaceae* (cypresses)
April-June	G	*Gramineae*
	G	*Poaceae*
July-August	W	*Ambrosia* (ragweed)
	C	*Humulus* (hops)
July-September	S	*Artemisia* (mugwort)
August-September	T	*Plantago* (plantains)
	W	*Chenopodiaceae* (goosefoot)
	W	*Urtica* (nettles)

AUSTRALIA – WESTERN AUSTRALIA

MONTH		PLANT NAME
May-February	T	*Acacia* (wattles)
July-November	T	*Casuarina* (she-oak or 'Australian pine')
	T	*Pinaceae* (pines)
	W	*Arctotheca calendula* (capeweed)
August-February	T	*Plantago* (plantains)
August-October	T	*Callitris columellaris* (white cypress pine)
	T	*Cupressaceae* (cypresses)
August-November	S	*Ligustrum* (privet)
September-January	W	*Rumex* (docks and sorrels)
September-February	W	*Chenopodiaceae* (goosefoots)
September-March	G	*Gramineae*
	G	*Poaceae*
October-February	C	*Helianthus* (sunflower)
October-March	T	*Eucalyptus* (gum trees)
October-November	W	*Echium plantagineum* (Peterson's curse or Salvation Jane)
November-December	T	*Olea* (olive trees)

AUSTRALIA – NORTHERN TERRITORY

MONTH		PLANT NAME
October-March	G	*Gramineae*
	G	*Poaceae*

AUSTRALIA – QUEENSLAND

MONTH		PLANT NAME
January-December	T	*Eucalyptus* (gum trees)
May-October	T	*Acacia* (wattles)
August-March	T	*Plantago* (plantains)
September-February	T	*Casuarina* (she-oak or 'Australian pine')
	W	*Rumex* (docks and sorrels)
September-April	W	*Chenopodiaceae* (goosefoots)

September-May	G	*Gramineae*
	G	*Poaceae*
September-November	S	*Ligustrum* (privet)
	T	*Callitris columellaris* (white cypress pine or Murray pine)
October-November	W	*Arctotheca calendula* (capeweed)
December-May	C	*Helianthus* (sunflower)

AUSTRALIA – NEW SOUTH WALES

MONTH		PLANT NAME
January-December	T	*Eucalyptus* (gum trees)
June-February	T	*Plantago* (plantains)
June-April	W	*Parietaria judaica* (pellitory-of-the-wall)
June-December	T	*Acacia* (wattles)
July-April	T	*Casuarina* (she-oak or 'Australian pine')
August-May	G	*Gramineae*
	G	*Poaceae*
August-November	T	*Callitris columellaris* (white cypress pine or Murray pine)
August-November	T	*Cupressaceae* (cypresses)
September-February	W	*Rumex* (docks and sorrels)
September-October	T	*Betula pendula* (silver birch)
September-November	S	*Ligustrum* (privet)
	W	*Arctotheca calendula* (capeweed)
September-December	W	*Echium plantagineum* (Paterson's curse or Salvation Jane)
October-November	T	*Olea* (olive trees)
December-January	W	*Artemisia* (wormwood)
December-February	W	*Chenopodiaceae* (goosefoots)
December-May	C	*Helianthus* (sunflower)

AUSTRALIA – VICTORIA

MONTH		PLANT NAME
January-December	T	*Eucalyptus* (gum trees)
March-April	T	*Casuarina* (she-oak or 'Australian pine')
April-September	T	*Cupressaceae* (cypresses)
June-October	T	*Callitris columellaris* (white cypress pine or Murray pine)
July-January	T	*Acacia* (wattles)
July-August	T	*Casuarina*
August-February	W	*Rumex* (docks and sorrels)
August-September	T	*Pinaceae* (pines)
August-December	W	*Arctotheca calendula* (capeweed)
	W	*Echium plantagineum* (Paterson's curse or Salvation Jane)
September-February	W	*Trifolium* (clover)
September-May	G	*Gramineae*
	G	*Poaceae*
September-October	T	*Betula pendula* (silver birch)
October-March	T	*Plantago* (plantains)
October-November	T	*Olea* (olive trees)
October-December	S	*Ligustrum* (privet)
December-April	W	*Chenopodiaceae* (goosefoots)

AUSTRALIA – SOUTH AUSTRALIA

MONTH		PLANT NAME
March-July	T	*Casuarina* (she-oak or 'Australian pine')
July-March	G	*Gramineae*
July-March	G	*Poaceae*
July-November	T	*Acacia* (wattles)
July-December	W	*Echium plantagineum* (Paterson's curse or Salvation Jane)
August-March	T	*Eucalyptus* (gum trees)
	T	*Plantago* (plantains)
August- September	T	Casuarina (she-oak or 'Australian pine')
August-October	T	*Callitris columellaris* (white cypress pine or Murray pine)
	T	*Cupressaceae* (cypresses)
August-November	W	*Arctotheca calendula* (capeweed)
September-February	W	*Trifolium* (clover)
September-November	T	*Betula pendula* (silver birch)
	T	*Olea* (olive trees)
	S	*Ligustrum* (privet)
September-December	W	*Rumex* (docks and sorrels)
December-April	W	*Chenopodiaceae* (goosefoots)

AUSTRALIA – TASMANIA

MONTH		PLANT NAME
June-December	T	*Casuarina* (she-oak or 'Australian pine')
July-November	T	*Cupressaceae* (cypresses)
	T	*Pinaceae* (pines)
August-February	T	*Acacia* (wattles)
	T	*Eucalyptus* (gum trees)
September-January	W	*Arctotheca calendula* (capeweed)
September-April	G	*Gramineae*
	G	*Poaceae*
September-May	W	*Rumex* (docks and sorrels)
September-November	T	*Betula pendula* (silver birch)
October-March	T	*Plantago* (plantains)

NEW ZEALAND

MONTH		PLANT NAME
January-March	W	*Rumex* (docks and sorrels)
July-October	T	*Pinaceae* (pines)
July-November	T	*Cupressaceae* (cypresses)
August-October	T	*Betula* (birches)
	T	*Quercus* (oaks)
August-November	T	*Acacia* (wattles)
August-November	T	*Albizia* (mimosas)
October-February	G	*Gramineae*
	G	*Poaceae*
	T	*Plantago* (plantains)
October-March	S	*Ligustrum* (privet)

HAWAII

MONTH		PLANT NAME
January-December (except late December)	G	*Gramineae*
	G	*Poaceae*
January-April	T	Various native and introduced species especially:
	T	*Cryptomeria* (Japanese red cedar)
	T	*Eucalyptus* (gum trees)
May (mid)-December	W	Weeds

CANADA – ALASKA (USA) AND NORTH CANADA

MONTH		PLANT NAME
April-May	T	*Alnus* (alder)
	T	*Populus* (poplars)
	T	*Salix* (willows)
April-June	T	*Myrica gale* (bog myrtle or sweet gale)
May-June	T	*Betula* (birches)
May-September	G	*Gramineae*
	G	*Poaceae*

CANADA – NORTHEAST

This area covers northern Ontario, northern Quebec, Labrador and Newfoundland.

MONTH		PLANT NAME
April-June	T	*Myrica gale* (bog myrtle or sweet gale)
May-June	T	*Betula* (birches)
July	G	*Gramineae*
	G	*Poaceae*
July-August	T	*Pinaceae* (spruce, fir and larch)

CANADA – SOUTHEAST

This area covers southern Ontario, southern Quebec, New Brunswick and Nova Scotia.

MONTH		PLANT NAME
April	T	*Alnus* (alders)
April-May	T	*Fraxinus* (ash trees)
	T	*Populus* (poplars)
	T	*Salix* (willows)
April-June	T	*Morus* (mulberry)
	T	*Myrica gale* (bog myrtle or sweet gale)
May-June	T	*Acer* (maples)
	T	*Betula* (birches)
	T	*Carya* (hickories)
	T	*Celtis* (hackberries)
	T	*Fagus* (beeches)
	T	*Quercus* (oaks)
	T	*Ulmus* (elms)
	S	*Ligustrum* (privet)
May-August	G	*Gramineae*
	G	*Poaceae*
June-August	T	*Pinaceae* (pines and spruces)
July	T	*Tilia* (lindens and basswoods)
July-September	W	*Chenopodiaceae* (goosefoots, pigweed and 'Russian thistle')
July-October	T	*Plantago* (plantains)
August-September	W	*Ambrosia* (ragweeds)
	W	*Artemisia* (mugwort and wormwoods)

BRITISH COLUMBIA

MONTH		PLANT NAME
February-June	T	*Cupressaceae* (cypresses, junipers and 'cedars'
April-May	T	*Alnus* (alders)
	T	*Populus* (poplars)
	T	*Salix* (willows)
April-June	T	*Myrica gale* (bog myrtle or sweet gale)
May-June	T	*Acer* (maples)
	T	*Betula* (birches)
May-September	G	*Gramineae*
	G	*Poaceae*
August-September	W	*Ambrosia* (ragweeds)

GREAT PLAINS OF CANADA

This area covers Alberta, Saskatchewan and Manitoba.

MONTH		PLANT NAME
March-June	T	*Cupressaceae* (cypresses, junipers and 'cedars'
April-May	T	*Betula* (birches)
	T	*Populus* (poplars and quaking aspen)
April-June	T	*Myrica gale* (bog myrtle or sweet gale)
May	T	*Quercus* (oaks)
May-June	T	*Acer* (maples)
	T	*Ulmus* (elms)
May-August	G	*Gramineae*
	G	*Poaceae*
August-September	T	*Plantago* (plantains)
	W	*Ambrosia* (ragweeds)
	W	*Artemisia* (mugwort and wormwoods)
	W	*Chenopodiaceae* (goosefoots)

USA – WASHINGTON AND OREGON

MONTH		PLANT NAME
February-April	T	*Alnus* (alder)
March-May	T	*Cupressaceae* (cypresses, junipers and 'cedars')
	T	*Populus* (poplars)
	T	*Salix* (willows)
	T	*Sequoia* (coast redwood)
April-May	T	*Acer* (maples)
	T	*Betula* (birches)
	T	*Quercus* (oaks)
April-September	G	*Gramineae*
	G	*Poaceae*
May-September	W	*Rumex* (docks and sorrels)
May-November	T	*Plantago* (plantains)
June-October	W	*Amaranthaceae* (amaranths)
	W	*Chenopodiaceae* (goosefoots)
July-October	W	*Ambrosia* (ragweeds)

USA – CALIFORNIA

MONTH		PLANT NAME
January-September	W	*Urtica* (nettles)
January-October	T	*Acacia* (wattles and acacias)
January-December	W	*Rumex* (docks and sorrels)
February-April	T	*Fraxinus* (ash)
	T	*Quercus* (oaks)
	T	*Ulmus* (elms)
February-May	T	*Myrica* (Bayberry or wax myrtle)
	T	*Casuarina* (she-oak or 'Australian pine')
February-July	W	*Parietaria* (pellitories)
March-April	T	*Cryptomeria* (Japanese red cedar)
March-May	T	*Acer* (maples)
	T	*Broussonetia* (paper mulberry)
	T	*Carya* (hickories)
	T	*Juglans* (walnuts and pecans)
	T	*Morus* (mulberry)
March-June	S	*Ligustrum* (privet)
April-May	T	*Populus* (poplars)
April-October	G	*Gramineae*
	G	*Poaceae*
April-December	W	*Amaranthaceae* (amaranths)
	W	*Ambrosia* (ragweeds)
	W	*Chenopodiaceae* (goosefoots)
May-June	T	*Olea* (olive trees)
May-July	S	*Prosopis* (mesquite)
May-November	T	*Plantago* (plantains)
June-December	T	*Arecaceae* (palm trees)
July-September	W	*Artemisia* (sagebrush)
August-October	T	*Ulmus* (elms)
August-November	W	*Iva* (poverty weeds and marsh elders)
September-March	T	*Cupressaceae* (cypresses, junipers and 'cedars')
September-November	T	*Casuarina* (she-oak or 'Australian pine')
December-March	T	*Eucalyptus* (gum trees)
December-May	T	*Alnus* (alders)
	T	*Betula* (birches)

USA – MONTANA, IDAHO AND WYOMING

MONTH		PLANT NAME
January-February	T	*Cupressaceae* (cypresses)
February-April	T	*Alnus* (alders)
	T	*Carpinus* (hornbeams)
	T	*Corylus* (hazels)
	T	*Ostrya* (ironwood)
March-May	T	*Populus* (poplars)
	T	*Salix* (willows)
April-May	T	*Betula* (birches)
April-May	T	*Quercus* (oaks)
May-September	G	*Gramineae*
	G	*Poaceae*
May-November	T	*Plantago* (plantains)
	W	*Rumex* (docks and sorrels)
June-October	W	*Amaranthaceae* (amaranths)
	W	*Chenopodiaceae* (goosefoots)
August-September	W	*Ambrosia* (ragweeds)
	W	*Artemisia* (sagebrush)

USA – NEVADA, UTAH AND COLORADO

MONTH		PLANT NAME
January-March	T	*Cupressaceae* (cypresses, junipers and 'cedars'
March-October	G	*Gramineae*
	G	*Poaceae*
April-May	T	*Populus* (poplars)
May-September	W	*Rumex* (docks and sorrels)
June-October	W	*Amaranthaceae* (amaranths)
	W	*Chenopodiaceae* (goosefoots)
July-September	W	*Parietaria* (pellitories)
August-September	W	*Ambrosia* (ragweeds)

USA – ARIZONA AND NEW MEXICO

MONTH		PLANT NAME
February-March	T	*Fraxinus* (ash trees)
February-November	G	*Gramineae*
	G	*Poaceae*
March-September	W	*Rumex* (docks and sorrels)
April-October	W	*Amaranthaceae* (amaranths)
	W	*Chenopodiaceae* (goosefoots)
May-June	T	*Olea* (olive trees)
May-July	S	*Prosopia* (mesquite)
July-September	W	*Artemisia* (sagebrush)
August-September	W	*Ambrosia* (ragweeds)
	W	*Franseria* (bur ragweed)
September-March	T	*Cupressaceae* (cypresses, junipers and 'cedars')

USA – THE SOUTH

This area includes Texas, Louisiana, Mississippi and Alabama.

MONTH		PLANT NAME
January-April	T	*Celtis* (hackberries and sugarberries)
	T	*Ulmus* (elms)
February-May	T	*Acer* (maples)
March-April	T	*Myrica cerifera* (Southern bayberry or wax myrtle)
March-May	T	*Broussonetica* (paper mulberry)
	T	*Carya* (hickories and pecans)
	T	*Morus* (mulberries)
March-June	S	*Ligustrum* (privet)
March-December	G	*Gramineae*
	G	*Poaceae*
April-June	S	*Maclura* (hedgeplant or osage orange)
June-December	W	*Amaranthaceae* (amaranths)
	W	*Chenopodiaceae* (goosefoots)
July-November	W	*Ambrosia* (ragweeds)
August-October	T	*Celtis* (hackberries and sugarberries)
	T	*Ulmus* (elms)
August-November	T	*Baccharis halmilifolia* (groundsel bush or tree)
	W	*Iva* (marsh elders and dune elder)
September-March	T	*Cupressaceae* (junipers and 'cedars')

USA – SOUTH-CENTRAL STATES

This area includes Kansas , Oklahoma, Missouri and Arkansas.

MONTH		PLANT NAME
February-March	T	*Celtis* (hackberries and sugarberries)
		Fraxinus (ash)
February-May	T	*Acer* (maples)
March-April	T	*Myrica cerifera* (southern bayberry or wax myrtle)
March-May	T	*Betula* (birches)
	T	*Broussonetia papyrifera* (paper mulberry)
April-May	T	*Quercus* (oaks)
	S	*Maclura* (osage orange or hedgeplant)
April-October	W	*Amaranthaceae* (amaranths)
	W	*Chenopodiaceae* (goosefoots)
April-November	G	*Gramineae*
	G	*Poaceae*
May-September	W	*Rumex* (docks and sorrels)
May-November	T	*Plantago* (plantains)
July-September	W	*Artemisia* (sagebrush)
August-September	W	*Ambrosia* (ragweeds)

USA – KENTUCKY AND TENNESSEE

MONTH		PLANT NAME
January-March	T	*Cupressaceae* ('cedars' and junipers)
February-March	T	*Acer* (maples)
March-April	T	*Salix* (willows)
April-May	T	*Quercus* (oaks)
April-September	W	*Rumex* (docks and sorrels)
May-August	G	*Gramineae*
	G	*Poaceae*
May-November	T	*Plantago* (plantains)
August-October	W	*Ambrosia* (ragweeds)
	W	*Artemisia* (wormwoods)

USA – THE MID-WEST

This area includes North and South Dakota, Nebraska, Minnesota, Michigan, Wisconsin, Iowa, Indiana and Idaho.

MONTH		PLANT NAME
February-April	T	*Alnus* (alder)
	T	*Carpinus* (ironwood)
	T	*Corylus* (hazel)
	T	*Ostrya* (hornbeam)
March-April	T	*Populus* (poplars)
	T	*Salix* (willows)
	T	*Ulmus* (elms)
April-May	T	*Acer* (maples)
	T	*Betula* (birches)
	T	*Fraxinus* (ash trees)
	T	*Quercus* (oaks)
May-June	S	*Ligustrum* (privet)
May-July	G	*Gramineae*
	G	*Poaceae*
May-September	W	*Rumex* (docks and sorrels)

May-November	T	*Plantago* (plantains)
June-September	W	*Cannabis sativa* (hemp or cannabis)
June-October	W	*Amaranthaceae* (amaranths)
June-October	W	*Chenopodiaceae* (goosefoots)
July-September	W	*Parietaria* (pellitories)
	W	*Pilea* (clearweed)
	W	*Urtica* (nettles)
July-October	W	*Ambrosia* (ragweeds)

USA – THE NORTH EAST AND NEW ENGLAND

This area covers Maine, New Hampshire, Vermont, Massachusetts, Connecticut, Rhode Island, Pennsylvania, New York State, New Jersey, Delaware and Virginia.

MONTH		PLANT NAME
February-April	T	*Ulmus* (elms)
February-May	T	*Acer* (maples)
March-April	T	*Populus* (poplars)
	T	*Salix* (willows)
March-May	T	*Cupressaceae* ('cedars' and junipers)
April-May	T	*Alnus* (alder)
	T	*Betula* (birches)
	T	*Carpinus* (ironwood)
	T	*Corylus* (hazels)
	T	*Ostrya* (hornbeams)
	T	*Pinaceae* (pines)
	T	*Quercus* (oaks and beeches)
April-June	S	*Comptonia peregrina* (sweet fern)
April-July	T	*Myrica* (bayberry or wax myrtle)
May	T	*Fraxinus* (ash trees)
May-June	S	*Ligustrum* (privet)
May-July	G	*Gramineae*
	G	*Poaceae*
May-September	W	*Rumex* (docks and sorrels)
May-October	W	*Pilea* (clearwood)
	W	*Urtica* (nettles)
June-July	T	*Tilia* (lindens or basswoods)
June-August	T	*Plantago* (plantains)
June-October	W	*Amaranthaceae* (amaranths)
	W	*Chenopodiaceae* (goosefoots)
	W	*Parietaria* (pellitories)
July-October	W	*Ambrosia* (ragweeds)
August-October	W	*Iva* (marsh elders)

USA – THE SOUTHEAST STATES

This area includes North Carolina, South Carolina, Georgia and Florida.

MONTH		PLANT NAME
January-June	W	*Parietaria* (pellitories)
February-April	T	*Betula* (birches)
	T	*Casuarina* (she-oaks or 'Australian pines'
February-May	T	*Quercus* (oaks)
March-May	T	*Acer* (maples)
	T	*Populus* (poplars)
	T	*Salix* (willows)
	T	*Ulmus* (elms)
March-June	T	*Broussonetia papyrifera* (paper mulberry)
March-October	G	*Gramineae*
	G	*Poaceae*
April-May	T	*Carya* (hickories)
	T	*Juglans* (walnuts)
	S	*Maclura* (osaga orange or hedgeplant)
April-June	T	*Acoelorrhaphe wrightii* (everglades palm)
	T	*Albizia* (mimosa or silk tree)
	W	*Rumex* (docks and sorrels)
April-October	W	*Amaranthaceae* (amaranths)
	W	*Chenopodiaceae* (goosefoots)
May-June	S	*Ligustrum* (privet)
May-November	T	*Plantago* (plantains)
July-November	W	*Ambrosia* (ragweeds)
August-September	W	*Iva* (marsh elders and dune elder)
August-October	W	*Pilea* (clearweed)
	W	*Urtica* (nettles)
October-December	T	*Casuarina* (she-oaks or 'Australian pines'
	T	*Myrica* (bayberry or wax myrtle)
December-March	T	*Cupressaceae* ('cedars', cypresses and junipers)
	T	*Eucalyptus* (gum trees)
	T	*Taxodium* (bald 'cypress', or swamp 'cypress' and pond 'cypress')
December-June	T	*Pinaceae* (pines)

CARIBBEAN

MONTH		PLANT NAME
February-April	T	*Casuarina* (she-oaks or 'Australian pines')
March-June	W	*Urtica* (nettles)
April-May	T	*Broussonetia papyrifera* (paper mulberry)
June-July	G	*Gramineae*
	G	*Poaceae*
June-October	T	*Celtis* (sugarberry or hackberry trees)
October-March	G	*Gramineae*
	G	*Poaceae*
December-August	W	*Parietaria judaica* (pellitory-of-the-wall)

SOUTH AMERICA

In countries north of the equator, such as Venezuela.

MONTH		PLANT NAME
April-July	G	Grasses

NORTHERN BRAZIL

MONTH		PLANT NAME
October-December	G	Grasses

RIO DE JANEIRO

MONTH		PLANT NAME
December-March	G	Grasses

ECUADOR

MONTH		PLANT NAME
January-December	G	Grasses

PERU

MONTH		PLANT NAME
October-January	G	Grasses

ARGENTINA

MONTH		PLANT NAME
October-February	G	Grasses

Avoiding allergens in the home

You spend much of your life in your home, so it's well worth taking the trouble to make sure that it's an allergen-free area – as much as possible, that is, because in some cases it is extremely difficult to keep allergens out. Within limits, you can make sure that any foods to which you are allergic are kept our of the house (see pp. 106–107), and you can refuse to give house room to any chemicals, such as cosmetics or shampoo, that cause an allergic reaction. It's more difficult to ensure success when – as in the case of biological washing powders, which can trigger eczema in susceptible individuals – the allergen is ubiquitous, and almost impossible if you suffer from hayfever or asthma attacks that are triggered by allergens in the very air that we breathe.

Nevertheless, any steps that you take to reduce the number of allergens in your home are likely to reduce the chances of an allergic reaction. And this is especially true when the allergens in question are pollen, house-dust mite droppings and mould spores.

EXCLUDING POLLEN

The prime cause of hayfever is pollen, and it is also responsible for a large number of asthma attacks, so it makes sense to take every possible step to exclude pollen from your home. If you know the types of pollen to which you are allergic (see pp. 102–105), focus your efforts on the appropriate times of year when those pollens are in the atmosphere. Remember that the pollen count rises at certain times of the day and in certain weather conditions (see pp. 108–109), so keep your windows tightly shut during these times to minimize the amount that enters your home. Make the most of any rain to air your home thoroughly, or open your windows in the late evening – you may have to close them again at sunrise, though. Always keep your windows shut and stay inside if anyone is mowing the grass nearby, or during harvest time if you live in the country.

All the above may be good advice, but it is very difficult to follow in most family homes. However, there is a compromise: you should attempt to keep your bedroom and one other room free of pollen. Grains of pollen are larger than many other allergens, and settle to the ground quite quickly when the air is still, taking about seven minutes in an average house. You can take advantage of this fact by asking a friend who does not suffer from hayfever or pollen-induced asthma to sit in your chosen room for at least seven minutes with the door shut and vacuum the floor and soft furnishings and wet-wash the furniture. Your friend must then creep out of the room, making sure that he or she doesn't slam the door and create movement in the air.

AIR FILTERS

The trouble is that the presence of children and pets reduces the chances that this tactic will be successful, because they make it almost impossible to keep the air in your house still. If such cases, the answer may be to buy an air filter in order to sieve pollen from the air.

A number of different types of filter exist, but the best are HEPA filters (High Efficiency Particulate Air), which must remove 99.9 per cent of particles from the air to merit their description. However, it is important that you buy one powerful enough to 'clean' the air in a room the same size as yours four times an hour.

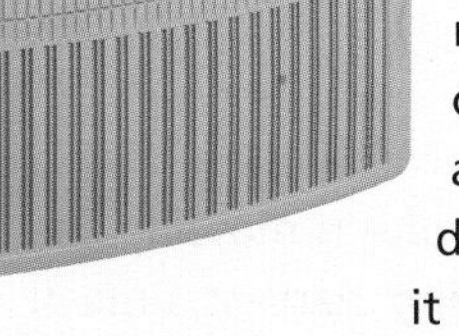

Air filter

MOULD SPORES

Cutting down on the movement of air is a good way of tackling the problem of pollen in the home, but it has annoying side-effect of increasing humidity. And warm, humid, still conditions are ones in which mould thrives – and mould spores can also cause hayfever or trigger asthma attacks. The answer is to use a dehumidifier that reduces the moisture from the air to under 45 per cent – some models can reduce moisture even further, but they should not be left on in a room in which someone is sleeping.

MITES

House-dust mites thrive in centrally heated, draught-free houses that have fitted carpets, heavy curtains and soft furnishings, and, like mould, they love humidity; they are also extremely tenacious. Their droppings can be responsible for hayfever attacks and can also trigger asthma attacks.

Apart from buying a humidifier, the obvious, though rather drastic solution to the problem of mites is to throw out all your carpets and have wooden floors, but if this is not feasible it is worth considering laying short-pile synthetic carpets. Hang cotton, washable curtains and wash them frequently at a high temperature (60°C/140°F) – you should fit washable covers on your chairs and sofas as well. Turn down the thermostat on your heating, and preferably leave your bedroom without heating.

Clean and vacuum your house regularly – at least twice a week – concentrating not just on the carpets but also on your bedding, soft furnishings and sofas. It is well worth buying a powerful vacuum that has a special allergen filter – ask your national allergy organization (see pp. 124–5) for a list of manufacturers and stockists. Mop floors wherever possible, but make sure that they dry quickly. Furniture should be wet-washed so that as much dust as possible is picked up, and then dried with a cloth to prevent water marks.

One of the main reservoirs of mites in your home is likely to be your bedding and mattress, because it is in bed that you shed much of your dead skin. High temperatures kill the mites, so at the very least it is sensible to choose bedding made from synthetic materials or cotton that can be washed at high temperatures (60°C/140°F or over) – dry cleaning them is not as effective. Wash linen and pillows weekly and duvets and blankets fortnightly. Alternatively, you can buy special dust-free and 'anti-allergy' duvets and covers that are non-toxic to humans but kill mites – contact your national allergy organization (see pp. 124–5) for addresses of stockists.

If neither of these options is possible, adopt the practice of airing your bedding by hanging it out of a window during the day – cold, dry weather is ideal, since the mites cannot survive in cold, dry air. You can also use cold as a weapon against mites by placing your pillows in a bag and placing them in your freezer overnight; the next day, wash them at a high temperature and follow with two hours in a hot drier.

A powerful vacuum cleaner fitted with a fine filter is essential in the fight against house-dust mites. Models that use a miniature tornado to create a powerful vacuum are much more effective than conventional models.

All these precautions will help to keep the population of mites down, but do not go to the root of the problem, which is likely to lie in your mattress. If funds allow, the best bet is to buy one of the new 'allergen-proof' covers, which are made from a microporous material that allows the mattress to breathe but prevents house-dust mite infestation – these are also less slippery and hot than plastic covers, and are stocked by most high-street pharmacists.

Otherwise, try treating your old mattress with acaricide (mites are more spiders than insects, and this is more effective than an insecticide). However, this treatment should not be undertaken by the person who suffers from hayfever, because there is a risk of a cross-reaction to it (see pp. 14–15). (Liquid nitrogen can also be used to kill of the mites, but this is the province of an outside specialist.) Afterwards, the room and all its contents must be vacuumed thoroughly to remove both the dead mites and their droppings.

PETS

Many people find that bouts of hayfever and asthma attacks are caused by the presence of cats and dogs. It's often thought that animal hair is responsible, but this is not, in fact, the case. The culprits are tiny particles of skin, and also of dried saliva, which is released into the atmosphere when an animal – a cat, in particular – grooms itself. Vacuuming with a machine that has a special filter will help remove these particles, as will air filters, but saliva tends to be particularly durable. Unfortunately, most people who suffer from hayfever or asthma as a result of pet saliva or skin particles find eventually that they can only keep a pet at the risk of further attacks.

IONIZERS

So far we have been discussing practical measures to control allergens, all of which take a great deal of time and trouble. However, there may be a simpler way: to buy an ionizer. This is certainly something that you should consider, because research undertaken at the University of Surrey found that 70 per cent of people using ionizers said that their hayfever had been helped.

The principle of ionization is fairly straightforward. The air that we breathe contains electrically charged particles that carry either a positive or negative charge, and these charged particles are known as 'ions'. In the countryside, there is normally a balance between the charges, although there are more positive ions in the air during certain weather conditions – when there is a warm, dry wind, for example. But in cities and towns pollution, dust and fumes can eliminate the negative ions in the air, and the ratio can fall from to one negative ion to three positive ions.

Ionizer

It has been found that a preponderance of positive ions in the air makes people feel irritable and bad-tempered, increases the incidence of general malaise and headaches and worsens symptoms of hayfever and asthma. You may have experienced the feeling yourself before a storm, when people often feel lethargic and depressed, as negative ions are reduced; after the storm has broken they feel invigorated. This is because negative ions are formed around moving water, such as rainstorms, waterfalls, rivers and the sea.

Ionizers emit negative ions into the atmosphere, and so freshen the air by increasing the proportion of negative ions to positive ions. But they can also attract and remove dust, smoke and pollen particles from the air, and so many of its allergens. And there is a physiological reason why they work, too: when the air is rich in allergens and positive ions, the cilia – hair-like filters in the nasal passages – become almost stationary; but negative ions increase their mobility, so that they can move the allergens away from the sensitive nasal passages and prevent inflammation; negative ions also have an anti-histamine effect (see pp. 10–11), and quite large reductions in blood histamine levels have been found after the use of an ionizer.

If you try an ionizer, you should persevere with it for at least two months, because some people find that it takes time to help. And it has to be said that ionizers do not always work – some people find them no help at all.

Avoiding allergens in the environment

Fresh air and sunshine are usually thought to be both healthy and enjoyable. But allergic people need to treat both with care. The best place for most allergy sufferers is the seaside. Levels of pollen and atmospheric pollutants are low, and sunlight and sea water are usually beneficial for eczema. Most allergy-sensitive people, however, have to live in more polluted areas. It is important, therefore, to take precautions when you are outdoors.

As usual, avoidance is the best policy. If at all possible, don't leave your house or workplace at times when there is a high pollen count or when air quality is poor. Remember that pollen counts are higher on warm, dry days, and tend to peak in the early evening. Conversely, pollen counts will be lower after rain.

You should also try to avoid any substance that may cause a cross-reaction (see pp. 14–15), though this can be particularly difficult if you live in an urban or industrialized area with a high level of atmospheric pollution. Sulphur dioxide and acid droplets are emitted from factories and power stations, and exhaust fumes from motor vehicles contain nitrogen oxides and ozone, all of which are harmful to those with respiratory allergies. Diesel fumes contain fine particulates, which are a common trigger for cross-reactions, so avoid taxis, lorries and buses, all of which run on diesel – especially during the heavy traffic of the morning or evening rush hour or when air quality is poor. One of the most common of outdoor pursuits is gardening, and there are special allergen avoidance

MEDICAL ALERT

If you are sensitive to insect stings, and are at risk of anaphylactic shock (see pp. 24–5), always take the following precautions:

- *check the inside of your car before driving off and keep the windows closed;*
- *take care when eating outdoors that you do not leave food lying around that might attract wasps and other insects;*
- *carry your emergency treatment kit with you at all times;*
- *wear a medical tag or bracelet identifying your condition.*

techniques that you can follow in the garden, in addition to those given here (see pp. 122–3).

SELF-PROTECTION

If you do have to leave the house at a time when the risk of exposure to allergens is high, there are various precautions you can take. Those who suffer from hayfever and allergic conjunctivitis often find that it helps to wear glasses to prevent pollen and other allergens from reaching the surface of the eye. Ordinary glasses or sunglasses offer some protection, but pollen can easily get around the sides. An alternative is to buy a pair of prescription glasses if you use them, or sunglasses or ones with plain glass in them if not, that have enclosed sides. Most opticians will be able to supply these.

There are also specialized spectacles in which a miniature battery-operated pump creates a flow of air between the glass and the eyes, thus keeping pollen at bay. However, these are considerably more expensive than more conventional models.

Obviously, enclosed glasses offer no protection against allergens that enter your body through your nose and mouth. For this, you will need to wear a mask that covers the nose and mouth as well as glasses to cover the eyes. This may look unwieldly, and is hardly fashionable, but most allergy sufferers find that they only need to wear them at times of particularly high risk, such as when walking or driving along heavily congested roads, or during the rush hour, or during harvest time or peak pollen season in rural areas. Three different types of mask are available, and it is important that you choose the correct one. First, there is the 'nuisance dust mask', which can filter out chemical irritants, pollen and other large particles, but not pollen fragments or smaller allergens. These can be bought at most pharmacists and health stores. Second, there is the simple dust mask used by builders, decorators and do-it-yourself enthusiasts, which can be obtained from builder's merchants and DIY stores. This filters out fine particles, but not chemical irritants such as diesel fumes. The third and best type of mask is the 'dust respirator'. This filters out chemical irritants and allergens down to a very small size, but they are more expensive. Contact your national allergy organization (see pp. 124–5) for more information on manufacturers and stockists of both masks and specialized eye-protectors.

AVOIDING ALLERGIES AWAY FROM HOME

If you have to leave home for any reason when the risk of exposure to allergens is high, take the following precautions:

- *wear protective spectacles and/or a face mask;*
- *wrap a scarf round your face on cold days;*
- *avoid long grass on warm summer days and keep car windows closed;*
- *avoid vigorous activity when the weather is cold.*

Avoiding allergens in the garden

The garden is rich in allergens. Not only is it an obvious source of pollen, but it often harbours moulds, stinging insects, irritant plants and a variety of chemical fertilizers and pesticides, all of which can trigger a response in sensitive people. While it is impossible to make your garden an allergen-free zone – even if you don't grow plants to whose pollen you are allergic, for example, you cannot prevent your neighbours from doing so – it is still sensible to take whatever precautions you can.

General hygiene is important in the garden of an allergic person. Make sure there are no untidy areas of wilderness, and use weed-killer to keep weeds at bay. If you have sensitive skin, always wear gloves when handling garden chemicals. Don't wear rubber or latex gloves, because they have been known to cause severe allergic reactions. Cotton gloves, or gloves with a cotton lining are best. Don't allow leaf litter to accumulate, although disposing of garden rubbish can also be a problem. Compost heaps can encourage mould formation and a bonfire can cover a large area with allergenic particles. Instead, bag grass cuttings and other garden rubbish, seal the bags and take them – or persuade someone else to take them – to the local waste site.

DESIGNING A LOW-RISK GARDEN

For many people, grass pollen is one of the main causes of allergic symptoms, and it is the lawn that is the prime source. If you are allergic to grass pollen, there are several measures you can take. One option is to take up the lawn and lay paving stones, but if this is not possible, you should make sure that the grass is cut frequently and kept short. You will need to be vigilant. Grass adapts to being cut short, and over time it learns to flower – which is when it produces pollen – closer and closer to the ground. Have the lawn cut – and edged, too – as soon as you see signs that it may be starting to flower. You should never mow your lawn yourself if you suffer from pollen-induced asthma or hayfever, even if it is not flowering, because cutting releases small allergens that are similar to grass pollen and lead to a cross-reaction (see pp. 14–`15).

Garden flowers are rarely the direct cause of asthma or hayfever, since they are pollinated by insects rather than by wind, and they are therefore rarely the source of wind-borne pollen. But they may be capable of causing a cross-reaction if they are from the same botanical family as the plants that produce pollen to which you are allergic. Look in a botanical book to check which plants are close relatives of the ones that cause you problems. In general, though, people with allergies should avoid planting ornamental grasses, or flowers in the daisy family, such as chrysanthemums, marigolds, asters and sunflowers. People who are allergic to ragweed should not plant goldenrod (*Solidago*). If you are allergic to insect stings, do not plant clumps of flowering plants, which will attract the enthusiastic attention of bees and wasps, and never go round the garden in bare feet. Certain plants – including poison ivy, ragweed, primulas, chrysanthemums and celery – are also known to cause eczema and other allergic symptoms, and should be avoided by sensitive people. Remember too that it is fairly easy for allergens to be transferred from the garden into the home. Pollen, for example, can settle easily into the coat of the family dog, and regular brushing and washing is necessary.

Tree pollen is another common cause of allergic reactions. If you have any choice in the matter avoid birches, willows, alders and hazels, whose catkins are abundant sources of wind-borne pollen in spring and early summer. Take care, too, that you don't bring them into the house to put into flower arrangements. Sometimes hedges that contain cypresses can cause problems, in which case the cypresses should be cut down and replaced with other shrubs, or even a wooden fence.

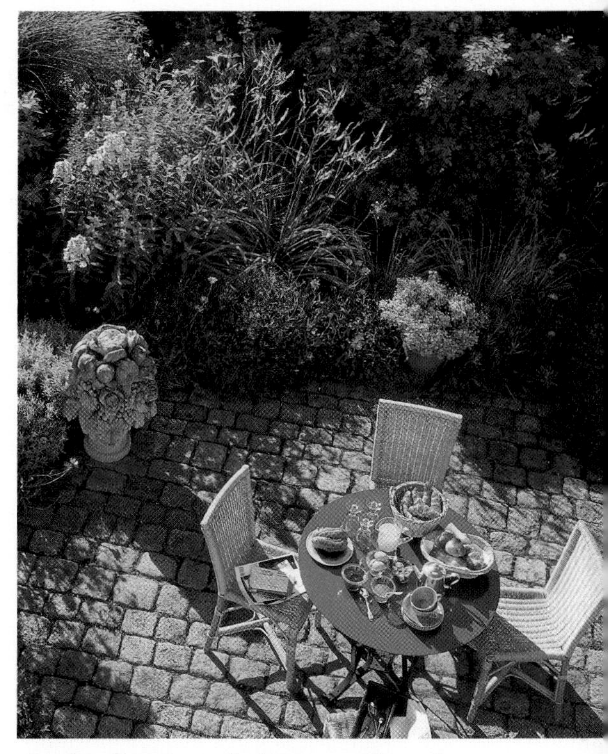

Garden flowers and plants pose less of a threat to hayfever sufferers than wildflowers and meadowgrasses, but certain species are to be avoided.

It may seem rather drastic to redesign your entire garden round an allergen-avoidance policy. However, the benefits in terms of reduced frequency and severity of allergic attacks – whether of asthma, hayfever, eczema or hives – more than outweigh the effort involved. And, in general terms, gardening provides an opportunity for some gentle exercise, as well as the opportunity to grow fruit and vegetables that will be free of potentially allergenic additives and other chemicals.

Useful addresses

The organizations listed here will offer practical help and advice on treating and coping with allergies, and include sources of information on a wide range of complementary and natural therapies.

GENERAL

United Kingdom
Action Against Allergy (AAA)
43 The Downs
London SW20 8HG
Tel: 44 181 947 5082

The Chi Centre
Riverbank House
Putney Bridge Approach
Fulham
London SW6 3JD
Tel: 44 171 371 9717

Food & Chemical Allergy Association
c/o The Chairman
Mrs Ellen Rathera
27 Ferringham Lane
Ferringham
West Sussex B12 5NB
Tel: 44 01903 41178

National Asthma Campaign
Providence House
Providence Place
London N1 0NT
Tel: 44 171 226 2260
Helpline: 44 0345 010203

The Asthma Society
Friends of the Asthma Research Council
300 Upper Street
London N2 X4
Tel: 44 171 226 2260

National Eczema Society
Tavistock House North
Tavistock Square
London WC1H 9SR
Tel: 44 171 388 4097

National Society for Research into Allergy
PO Box 43
Hinckley
Leicestershire LE10 1JY

The British Allergy Foundation
Helpline: 0891 516500

Register of Chinese Herbal Medicine
PO Box 400
Wembley
Middlesex HA9 9NZ
Tel: 44 181 904 1357

Society for Environmental Therapy
3 Atherton Road
Ipswich
Suffolk IP4 2LD

British Society for Allergy and Clinical Immunology
56 New Cavendish Street
London W1M 7RE
Tel: 44 171 486 0531

British Complementary Medicine Association
St Charles Hospital
Exmoor Street
London W10 6DZ
Tel: 44 181 964 1205

Yoga for Health Foundation
Ickwell Bury
Biggleswade
Bedfordshire
SG198 9EF
Tel: 44 176 727 271

ACUPUNCTURE

United Kingdom
British Acupuncture Council
Park House
206-208 Latimer Road
London W10 6RE
Tel: 44 181 964 0222

North America
American Association for Acupuncture
4101 Lake Boone Trail
Suite 201
Raleigh
North Carolina 27607
USA
Tel: 001 919 787 5181

New Zealand
New Zealand Register of Acupuncturists
PO Box 9950
Wellington 1
New Zealand
Tel: 64 4 476 8578

ALEXANDER TECHNIQUE

United Kingdom
Society of Teachers of the Alexander Technique
20 London House
266 Fulham Road
London SW10 9EL
Tel: 44 171 351 0828

North America
North American Society of Teachers of the Alexander Technique
PO Box 517
Urbana
Illinois 61801-0517
USA
Tel: 001 217 367 6956

Canadian Society of Teachers of the Alexander Technique
PO Box 47025
19-555 West 12th Avenue
Vancouver
British Columbia V5Z 3 XO
Canada

Australia
Australian Society of Teachers of the Alexander Technique
PO Box 716
DarlinghurstNew South Wales 2010
Australia
Tel: 61 8339 571

AROMATHERAPY

United Kingdom
International Federation of Aromatherapists
Stamford House
2-4 Chiswick High Road
London W4 1TH
Tel: 44 181 742 2605

North America
American Aromatherapy Association
PO Box 3679
South Pasadena
California 91031
USA
Tel: 001 818 457 1742

FLOWER REMEDIES

United Kingdom
Dr Edward Bach Centre
Mount Vernon
Sotwell
Wallingford
Oxon OX10 0PZ
Tel: 44 1491 834678

International Federation of Vibrational Medicine
Middle Piccadilly
Holwell
Dorset DT9 5LW
UK
Tel: 44 1963 23038

North America
Dr Edward Bach Healing Society
644 Merrick Road
Lynbrook
New York
USA
Tel: 001 516 593 2206

Australia
Martin & Pleasance
137 Swan Street
Richmond
Victoria 3121
Australia
Tel: 61 39 427 7422

HERBALISM

United Kingdom
School of Herbal Medicine
Bucksteep Manor
Bodle Street Green
Near Hailsham
Sussex BN27 4RJ
Tel: 44 1323 833 812/4

North America
American Herbalists Guild
PO Box 1683
Soquel
California 95073
USA

Australia
National Herbalists Association of Australia
Suite 305
BST House
3 Smail Street
Broadway
New South Wales 2007
Australia
Tel: 61 2 211 6437

HOMEOPATHY

United Kingdom
British Homeopathic Association
27A Devonshire Street
London W1N 1RJ
Tel: 44 171 935 2163

North America
National Center for Homeopathy
801 N Fairfax Street
Alexandria
VA 22314
USA
Tel: 001 703 548 7790

HYDROTHERAPY

Europe
UK College of Hydrotherapy
515 Hagley Road
Birmingham B66 4AX
Tel: 44 121 429 9191

North America
Aquatic Exercise Association
PO Box 1609
Nokomis
Florida 34274
USA
Tel: 001 813 486 8600

HYPNOTHERAPY

United Kingdom
British Hypnotherapy Association
67 Upper Berkeley Street
London
W1H 7DH
Tel: 44 171 723 4443

North America
American Association of Professional Hypnotherapists
PO Box 29
Boones Mill
Virginia 24065
USA
Tel: 001 703 334 3035

MASSAGE

United Kingdom
British Massage Therapy Council
Greenbank House
65a Adelphi Street
Preston PR1 7BH
Tel: 44 1772 881 063

North America
National Association of Massage Therapy
PO Box 1400
Westminster
Colorado 80030-1400
USA
Tel: 001 800 776 6268

Australia
Association of Massage Therapists
18a Spit Road
Mosman
New South Wales
Australia
Tel: 02 969 8445

NATUROPATHY

United Kingdom
General Council and Register of Naturopaths
Goswell House
Goswell Road
Street
Somerset BA16 0JG
Tel: 44 1458 840072

North America
American Association of Naturopathic Physicians
PO Box 20386
Seattle
Washington 98102
USA
Tel: 001 205 323 7610

Canadian Naturopathic Association
205, 1234 17th Avenue
South West
PO Box 4143
Station C
Calgary
Alberta
Canada
Tel: 001 413 244 4487

North American Society of Teachers of the Alexander Technique
PO Box 517
Urbana
Illinois 61801-0517
USA
Tel: 001 217 367 6956

Canadian Society of Teachers of the Alexander Technique
PO Box 47025
19-555 West 12th Avenue
Vancouver
British Columbia V5Z 3 XO
Canada

Australia
Australian Society of Teachers of the Alexander Technique
PO Box 716
Darlinghurst
New South Wales 2010
Australia
Tel: 61 8339 571

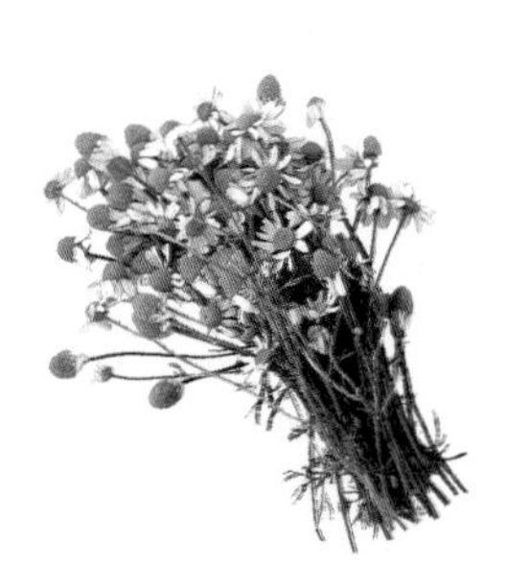

Index

Page numbers in italics refer to captions to illustrations